Streptokinase in Chronic Arterial Disease

Author
Michael Martin, M.D.
Professor of Medicine
Head, Geriatric Department
Municipal Hospital
Duisburg, West Germany

Technical Supervision

H. Auel

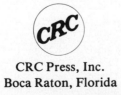

CRC Press, Inc.
Boca Raton, Florida

Library of Congress Cataloging in Publication Data

Martin, Michael, 1932-
    Streptokinase in chronic arterial disease.

    Bibliography: p.
    Includes index.
    1. Arterial occlusions—Chemotherapy.
2. Streptokinase—Therapeutic use. 3. Arteries—
Stenosis—Chemotherapy. 4. Chronic diseases—
Chemotherapy. I. Title.
RC694.3.M37   616.1'35061   81-15530
ISBN 0-8493-5046-8   AACR2

    Direct all inquiries to CRC Press, Inc., 2000 Corporate Blvd., N.W., Boca Raton, Florida, 33431.

© 1982 by CRC Press, Inc.

International Standard Book Number 0-8493-5046-8

Library of Congress Card Number 81-15530
Printed in the United States

PREFACE

Until 1967 a general belief was persistent among physicians working in the fields of angiology and blood coagulation that chronic arterial occlusions older than 6 days could not be dissolved by fibrinolytic treatment. Therefore, when on December 14, 1967, the first chronic femoral occlusion of 10 months standing and on February 22, 1968, the first iliac chronic occlusion of 3 months standing were removed by strepto-kinase treatment, our group was filled with enthusiasm and compared this result with the historical event of the first manned lunar orbiting by Apollo 8, which was carried out during that period (December 21, 1968). At that time, we envisioned a thrombol-ytic treatment of the obliterative disease as safe and technically perfect in its way as that of the lunar experiment. However, we learned soon enough that this goal was not easily reached, and that a lot of preparatory work still had to be done. The following chapters deal with these basic and tentative steps.

Michael Martin
Duisburg
October 1, 1981

THE AUTHOR

Michael Martin, M.D., is Professor of Medicine at the University of Bonn and holds the position as Head of Geriatric Department of the Municipal Teaching Hospital at Duisburg, West Germany.

Dr. Martin both graduated from and received his M.D. degree from the University of Hamburg.

From 1963 to 1977 Dr. Martin had his postgraduate training at the Anatomical Institute in Freiburg/Breisgau, at the Aggertalklinik, Clinic of Vascular Diseases, in Engelskirchen — Cologne and at the Medical Department of the University Hospital in Bonn. Dr. Martin has been Head of the Geriatric Department in Duisburg since 1977.

Dr. Martin's areas of specialization and interest include Internal Medicine with a special view to geriatrics, vascular diseases, blood coagulation disorders, and fibrinolytic treatment.

The list of professional societies to which Dr. Martin belongs includes Deutsche Gesellschaft fur Gerontologie, British Geriatric Society, American Geriatric Society, Canadian Association on Gerontology, Deutsche Arbeitsgemeinschaft fur Blutgerinnungsforschung, and Deutsche Gesellschaft fur Angiologie.

Dr. Martin has authored more than 100 papers on angiology, blood coagulation, fibrinolysis and geontology. He also authored a book (together with W. Schoop and E. Zeitler) *Thrombolytic Treatment of Chronic Arterial Occlusions* (in German). He edited two symposia, *New Concepts in Streptokinase Dosimetry* and on *Defibrination with Snake Venom Enzymes.* Dr. Martin translated the book *Geriatrics for Students* by Brocklehurst and Hanley. He is also on the International Advisory Board of *Age and Ageing* (London).

ACKNOWLEDGMENTS

The very first stimulation for conducting streptokinase treatment on patients displaying various forms of chronic obliterative disease came from the experimental work of H. Rosolleck and R. Gottlob who independently showed that chronic occlusion masses were easily resolved by streptokinase. In 1967, W. Schoop, head of the Aggertalklinik, D. Zekorn, Research Director of Behringwerke, E. Zeitler, head of the Radiology Department of the Aggertalklinik, and I were convinced that enough evidence was at hand for initiating a clinical trial of streptokinase treatment. Therapeutic work was started immediately thereafter, aimed at resolving chronic arterial obstruction in patients suffering from severe forms of the obliterative disease.

It seems difficult, if not impossible, to mention all colleagues, nurses, and technicians participating in the study. Virtually the whole staff of the Aggertalklinik worked, either for a short period or longer, in one way or another, in the fibrinolytic field. However, I wish to make special mention of some colleagues. First of all, I would like to name the head of the Aggertalklinik, Professor Schoop, who not only gave the very first stimulation to the fibrinolytic work, the results of which are accumulated in this study, but who also took an active part in the work by giving valuable advice and setting up tough and standardized criteria for the interpretation of clinical results.

Next, I wish to thank Professor Eberhard Zeitler who, as head of Radiology, provided us with hundreds of pre- and post-treatment angiograms. From the very beginning of the study, the angiographic proof of lytic results was regarded mandatory in order to introduce this new form of treatment to the scientific world. I look back with great pleasure at the lively relationship between our two departments (internal medicine, radiology) which deepened even more when a cooperative study of combined catheter recanalization (done by the radiologist) and fibrinolytic treatment (carried out by the internist) was launched. All angiograms shown in this book are furnished by Professor Zeitler's department and are presented here with his kind permission.

The following colleagues conducted and monitored streptokinase infusions at the bedside of a great number of patients. These were Dr. F. Aboudan, Dr. W. Blickle, Dr. G. Blumm, Dr. C.-D. Bluschke, Dr. J. Bopp, Dr. U. Buchner, Dr. H.-J. Engelken, Dr. R. Honnet, Dr. H. Mansjoer, Dr. J. Reichhold, Dr. I. Schmidtke, Dr. F. Tambert and Dr. C. Theobald. Three of them, Dr. Bluschke, Dr. Buchner and Dr. Engelken, defended their theses dealing with special problems of streptokinase therapy at the University of Bonn and, without exception, proceeded to obtain their doctoral degrees.

Next, I have been singularly fortunate in relying on a well functioning coagulation laboratory headed by Mrs. E. Perscheid and Mrs. I. Auras, both of whom provided us with a great variety of coagulation and fibrinolysis data.

Apart from these routine investigations, Sister Maria Hedwig, Mrs. B. Heimann, Mrs. R. Albrecht and Mrs. M. Altmaier were doing scientific work in my private laboratory at the Aggertalklinik in Engelskirchen as well as at the University Hospital in Bonn with a view to developing new methods for monitoring fibrinolytic treatment.

Additionally, Mrs. L. Blattner and Mr. H. Knoop were responsible for recording fibrinolytic results by means of oscillography and ultra sound Doppler measurements. Furthermore, Mrs. Blattner was in charge of the photo-lab and in this function provided us with graphic and angiographic reproductions.

I have a special debt to Mrs. Elinor Rathje who not only typed and retyped the whole series of chapters, but also led me, with patience and good humor, through the task of writing a book in a language not of my own tongue.

Doing the theoretical and practical work presented here and molding it into the form of a monograph are expensive ventures likely to remain uncompleted due to monetary reasons. Fortunately, however, I was able to rely on funds of the Verein zur Bekämpfung der Gefäßkrankheiten e.V., Engelskirchen, a nonprofit organization aimed at providing means for scientific research in the field of vascular diseases.

TABLE OF CONTENTS

Chapter 1

SCOPE OF THE STUDY*

The present study reports on 600 streptokinase infusion series. Major targets of treatment were arterial occlusions (most of them chronic) and arterial narrowings of the lower limbs. The clinical part of this survey will restrict itself entirely to these vascular areas. The average patient age was 53.7 years for 554 men (range 24 to 71 years) and 54.7 years for 46 women (28 to 78 years).

Eleven patients were treated for 1 day or less, 128 patients for 2 or 2.5 days, 447 patients for 3 days, and 14 patients for 4 days.

The streptokinase maintenance doses applied were 5000 u/hr in 10 patients, 30,000 u/hr in 17 patients, 100,000 u/hr in 568 patients (this includes 57 intermittent treatment series), and an escalating inflow scheme in 5 patients. Although it was quite nebulous (and in some ways unlikely) that this regimen would represent the most effective one, we held that administering a *uniform* streptokinase regimen to a *large* number of patients was the first step in providing a basis for further trials testing the efficiency of various different treatment forms.

At the beginning of the study a great number of basic questions connected with streptokinase therapy were still open; such as: how long was streptokinase stable in the infusion medium and at what intervals should new SK solutions be prepared? In the infusion medium, could streptokinase, known to decay under the influence of acids, be stored together with heparin which is described as a strong anionic compound? To what extent were current methods of anti-SK titer determination a reliable means for calculating the anti-SK neutralizing loading dose? Could the circulating anti-SK content be regarded as a parameter necessary for establishing the SK maintenance dose (SK influx per hour)? Was it advisable to calculate the streptokinase maintenance dose according to body weight?

In the following chapters some answers to the above questions are provided.

Last but not least, an urgent problem concerned the durability of lytic results. Streptokinase treatment would not be recommendable (even with a high thrombus removal rate) if clearance of an arterial segment lasted only a few months, i.e., if early reocclusion was the inevitable fate of each lytic effect. Therefore a six year retrospective investigation of the behavior of arteries, formerly occluded but later cleared by streptokinase treatment, was included as an integral part of this study.

* Some paragraphs in this chapter have been prepublished by M. Martin in *Prog. Cardiovasc. Dis.*, 21, 5, 1979. We thank Grune and & Stratton for the permission to reprint these items.

Chapter 2

CHARACTERISTICS OF PARTICIPANTS INVOLVED IN STREPTOKINASE TREATMENT

The seven main principles involved in fibrinolytic mechanisms are

- Plasminogen
- Plasmin
- Antiplasmin
- Streptokinase
- Activator
- Fibrinogen, Fibrin, Fibrinogen Degradation Products (FDP)
- Antistreptokinase

I. PLASMINOGEN

Plasminogen is a protein stable to acids but not to heat. In man, two slightly different plasminogen forms exist, namely, Glu-plasminogen and Lys-plasminogen (Summaria et al.[22]). In both cases the molecular weight is about 80,000. Plasminogen contains carbohydrate. In the electrophoresis it behaves like a beta globulin. Plasminogen is the inert precursor of the proteolytically active enzyme, plasmin. The precise tissue site of plasminogen synthesis has not been clearly elucidated. Barnhart and Riddle[2] have provided evidence indicating that the eosinophilic leukocytes may play a role. On the other hand, plasminogen concentration is low in the final stages of advanced hepatic diseases (as cirrhosis). Therefore, the liver cannot be excluded as a producer of plasminogen (Table 1). The biological variation of plasminogen values in a group of 65 men aged 40 to 65 years was calculated at $\pm 21\%$.

II. PLASMIN

The activated form of plasminogen is plasmin. The mechanism of Lys-plasminogen activation involves the cleavage of a sensitive arginyl-valine bond, thus leading to a two-chain molecule with a carboxymethyl heavy chain (A-chain) and a carboxymethyl light chain (B-chain), both of which are held together by a disulfide bridge.

Glu-plasminogen activation is accomplished by cleavage of the sensitive arginyl-valine peptide bond mentioned above, and by additional cleavage of a smaller peptide part (Robbins et al.[19]).

Plasmin is capable of splitting lysil-lysil or lysil-arginyl bonds contained in fibrinogen and fibrin. Furthermore, factors V and VIII, casein, gelatin, and protamine-heparin complex are digested by plasmin.

III. ANTIPLASMIN

The plasmin inhibitor concentration in human plasma far exceeds the corresponding plasmin activity. Recently it has become generally accepted to distinguish between a quick reacting antiplasmin "alpha-2-macroglobulin" and a progressive acting antiplasmin "alpha-1-antitrypsin". From the clinical point of view, the progressive antiplasmin seems to be the most important. As was shown by Nachman[16] the plasmin-progressive antiplasmin binding capacity depends on incubation time and temperature.

In 1975 Collen et al.[6] identified a fast-reacting plasmin inhibitor (α_2-antiplasmin)

Table 1
PLASMINOGEN CONCENTRATIONS IN PATIENTS DISPLAYING
DIFFERENT DISEASES

Disease	Plasminogen (%)
Renal hypertension	100
Visceral lupus erythematosus	100
Bronchial carcinoma	100
Rheumatoid arthrosis	100
Multiple myeloma	100
Arterial occlusive disease (Pat. No. 1)	100
Arterial occlusive disease (Pat. No. 2)	90
Arterial occlusive disease (Pat. No. 3)	100
Acute leukemia	100
Bilateral nephrectomy (Pat. No. 1)	100
Bilateral nephrectomy (Pat. No. 2)	100
Hepatic cirrhosis with coma (Pat. No. 1)	65
Hepatic cirrhosis (Pat. No. 2)	46
Hepatic cirrhosis (Pat. No. 3)	65

which they conceived as the most powerful plasmin inhibiting principle present in human plasma. In purified systems, and in plasma, α_2-antiplasmin forms a 1:1 stoichiometric complex with plasmin which is then devoid of protease or esterase activity and which cannot be dissociated with denaturating agents. Plasmin formed on the fibrin surface with its active sites involved in fibrin digestion reacts very slowly with α_2-antiplasmin. This specific interaction between plasmin, fibrin, and α_2-antiplasmin provide a molecular basis for the classical hypothesis which claims that plasminogen binds to fibrin and, following activation within the thrombus, exerts its action in a relatively inhibitor-free environment (Collen[5]).

Another antiplasmin, possibly of clinical importance, is antithrombin III. Heparin added to plasma combines with antithrombin III, thus establishing two major principles: first, an anticoagulant property widely used in antithrombotic prophylaxis; and second, a measurable activity of antiplasmin, the latter of which may possibly play a role during combined streptokinase-heparin infusion therapy (Telesforo et al.[24]).

IV. STREPTOKINASE

Streptokinase is a protein probably consisting of one chain of amino acids. The molecular weight is estimated to be about 50,000. There are no indications of streptokinase being a protease. This is one of many important differences in relation to urokinase, which splits lysine-arginine esters. In the electrophoresis, streptokinase behaves like an alpha-2-globulin.

Streptokinase is an exotoxin of beta hemolytic streptococci and can be isolated on a commercial basis with sufficient purity. In 1933, Tillet and Garner[25] were the first to provide evidence of the fibrinolytic effect of cultivated streptococci. The fibrinolytic active principle was called "streptococcal fibrinolysin". In 1945, Christensen and McLeod[4] held that streptokinase cannot be regarded as a protease but rather as a stimulator of proteolytic systems reacting in human blood. Consequently, they pleaded to have the term "streptococcal fibrinolysin" replaced by the more exact name, "streptokinase".

Low streptokinase concentrations in human plasma, as observed during streptokinase infusion, are relatively unstable, exerting a 20% fall during 1 hr storage at room temperature[1] (Figure 1). Streptokinase concentrations, as used for therapeutic purposes (1500 u/mℓ, 50,000 u/mℓ), are stable up to 48 hr irrespective of the solvent used. Heparin admixture to streptokinase does not reduce its stability.[12]

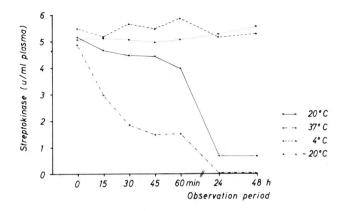

FIGURE 1. Decay rate of 5 u streptokinase added to 1 mℓ of anti-streptokinase-free plasma (post lysis plasma = plasma drawn 2 hr to 4 hr after discontinuation of SK infusion). The samples were stored at different temperatures (37°C, 20°C, 4°C, −20°C).

V. ACTIVATOR

Müllertz[15] was the first to give a more extensive explanation of the streptokinase effect on human plasma. He assumed a circulating "proactivator" substance which could easily be converted into "activator" by streptokinase. This activator was thought to convert plasminogen into the fibrinolytic enzyme plasmin.

In 1957 proof of this concept was established by Kline and Fishman[9]. They confirmed the assumption of Müllertz that plasminogen-plasmin conversion required a defined amount of proactivator and showed that plasminogen by itself could be looked upon as the proactivator substance. To date this view is accepted by most investigators. According to De Renzo[18], Heimburger and Schwick[7], Davis and Englebert,[6a] and Hummel et al.[8] one mole of streptokinase combines with one mole of plasminogen to form one mole activator.

According to Schwick[20] 1 mℓ of plasma contains 200 μg plasminogen. As 1μg plasminogen equals 1.1×10^{-11} mol, 1 mℓ of plasma will contain 220×10^{-11} mol plasminogen. Considering that 1 mol streptokinase stands for 5.17×10^{12} u streptokinase, then 220×10^{-11} mol streptokinase represent 11,500 u SK. These figures indicate that a 10,000 u SK/mℓ plasma mixture nearly represents an equimolar activator solution.

It was shown by Summaria et al.[22] that immediately after forming, the activator complex undergoes a typical sequence of changes. Plasminogen transforms within minutes into plasmin, whereas the streptokinase part splits into several degradation fragments, some of which still display streptokinase activity:

SK-plasminogen (activator) → SK-plasmin (activator)

The activator complex is subject to a certain degree of *dissociation*. It has been possible to demonstrate that in a 1:4320 diluted plasma containing equimolar components, more than 7/8 of both the streptokinase and the plasminogen molecules were present in their free form and available for further activator formation upon adding either a surplus of streptokinase or a surplus of plasminogen to the equimolar moiety.[11] When undiluted plasma was tested, an activator dissociation rate of about 50% was found, i.e., only about half of the streptokinase and plasminogen molecules were activator-bound, whereas the other half was circulating freely in the solution[13] (Figure 2).

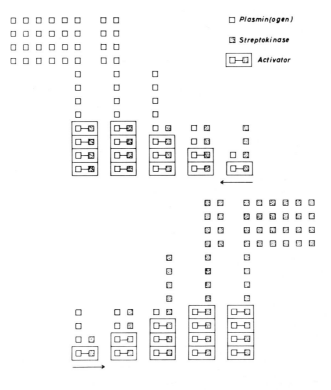

FIGURE 2. Schematic representation of the activator formation process. Upon mixing equal molarities of streptokinase and human plasminogen, only fractions of these reaction participants build up the activator complex. An ample number of molecules remain unbound and are at disposal for further activator formation.

VI. FIBRINOGEN, FIBRIN, FIBRINOGEN DEGRADATION PRODUCTS (FDP)

According to Blombäck and Blombäck[3] fibrinogen can be looked upon as a dimer consisting of one alpha, beta, and gamma chain each. The molecular weight is about 340,000. The chains are held together by disulfide bridges. One part of the molecule, called the "disulfide knot", plays an essential role in the studies of fibrinogen structure.

The conversion of fibrinogen into fibrin is performed by thrombin. The mechanism consists of splitting off fibrino-peptides A and B which, in turn, enables the molecules to form longitudinal and lateral (end-to-end and side-to-side) aggregates leading to the visible fibrin thread.

Fibrinogen, as well as fibrin, is susceptible to proteolytic actions of plasmin. The resulting split derivatives are fibrinogen/fibrin split products (FDP). According to Nussenzweig et al.[17] Latallo et al.[10] and Seligmann and Marder[21], fractions X, A, B, C, Y, D and E can be identified using electrophoretical methods and heating procedures (Figure 3). Fragment Y is a potent antithrombin, whereas fragment D acts mainly as inhibitor of fibrinogen monomer polymerization. Fragment E seems to be involved in inhibiting the thromboplastin generation. In 1970, a dialyzable component was described by Stachurska and co-workers[23] as being an inhibitor of thrombocyte aggregation and adhesion.

Fibrinogen /Fibrin - Degradation Products

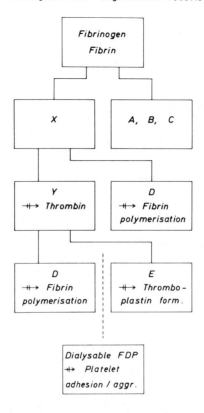

FIGURE 3. Schematic representation of fibrinogen degradation products (FDP) as determined during fibrinolytic treatment. Some of their possible effects on blood coagulation are indicated.

VII. ANTISTREPTOKINASE

Antistreptokinase is an antibody acquired against one of the exotoxins of streptococci. In the electrophoresis it runs as a gammaglobulin. Antistreptokinase titers can be measured by monitoring lysis times of whole blood clots coagulated with different amounts of streptokinase. The streptokinase concentration dissolving a defined clot within 10 min, multiplied by the patient's blood volume, is defined as "circulating anti-SK content" (CAC) and expressed in anti-SK units (method according to Deutsch and Fischer. See Chapter 16, Section III).

During recent years, various groups have reported a continuous fall in antistreptokinase values among patients. At the Aggertalklinik we have found a mean CAC of 252,000 ± 216,000 anti-SK units during 1968 (Figure 4). In contrast, the respective mean value for 1972 was 135,000 ± 117,000 anti-SK units. This corresponds to an overall decline of 40%. Likewise, in 1968 90% of our patients had a CAC below 550,000 anti-SK units, whereas in 1973 90% had a CAC below 250,000 anti-SK units. According to some authors, the steady decrease in CAC might be due to a concomitant fall in streptococcal infection rates under the influence of modern antibiotic treatment.

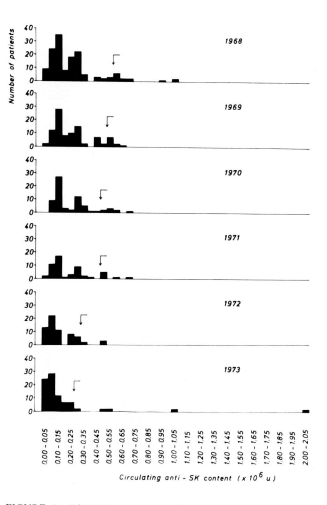

FIGURE 4. Distribution of circulating antistreptokinase contents (CAC) from 1968 through 1973. All determinations were carried out according to the method of Deutsch and Fischer 1960. A continuing decrease in CAC was found in the course of the years surveyed. For example, in 1968 90% of the patients tested had a CAC below 550,000 antistreptokinase units. By contrast, in 1973 90% displayed a CAC below 250,000 antistreptokinase units. ⌐ separates 90% (left side) and 10% (right side) of the respective patient groups.

REFERENCES

1. **Auel, H. and Martin, M.,** Die Technik des quantitativen Streptokinasenachweises, im *Plasma. Klin. Wschr.,* 53, 809, 1975.
2. **Barnhart, M. L. and Riddle, J. M.,** Cellular localization of profibrinolysin (plasminogen), *Blood,* 21, 306, 1963.
3. **Blombäck, M. and Blombäck, B.,** On the fibrinogen structure, Defibrinierung mit thrombinähnlichen Schlangengiftenzymen. VI. *Angiologisches Symposium der Aggertalklinik,* Martin, M. and Schoop, W., Eds., Verl. Hans Huber, Bern, 1975, 18.
4. **Christensen, L. R. and McLeod, C. M.,** A proteolytic enzyme of serum: characterization, activation, and reaction with inhibitors, *J. Gen. Physiol.,* 28, 559, 1945.

5. Collen, D., Inhibitors of fibrinolysis, in *Fibrinolysis*, Kline, D. L. and Reddy, K. N. N., Eds., CRC Press, Boca Raton, Fla., 1980, 130.

6. Collen, D., De Cock, F., and Verstraete, M., Immunochemical distinction between antiplasmin and antitrypsin, *Thromb. Res.*, 7, 245, 1975.

6a. Davies, M. C., Englebert, M. E. and De Renzo, E. C., Interaction of streptokinase and human plasminogen. I. Combining of streptokinase and plasminogen observed in the ultracentrifuge under a variety of experimental conditions, *J. Biol. Chem.*, 239, 265T, 1964.

7. Heimburger, N. and Schwick, H. G., Die Fibrinagarelektrophorese. 2. Mitteilung: Untersuchungen zum Wirkungsmechanismus der Streptokinase, *Thrombos. Diathes. haemorrh. (Stuttg.)*, 7, 444, 1962.

8. Hummel, B. C. W., Buck, F. F., and DeRenzo, E. C., Interaction of streptokinase and human plasminogen, *J. Biol. Chem.*, 241, 3474, 1966.

9. Kline, D. L. and Fishman, J. B., Plasmin: the humoral protease, *Ann. N.Y. Acad. Sci.*, 68, 25, 1957.

10. Latallo, Z. S., Budzinski, A. Z., Lipinski, B., and Kowalski, E., Inhibition of thrombin and of fibrin polymerization, two activities derived from plasmin-digested fibrinogen, *Nature (London)*, 203, 1184, 1964.

11. Martin, M., Studies on activator formation in human plasma with streptokinase. I. Experimental studies, *Thrombos. Diathes. haemorrh. (Stuttg.)*, 30, 381, 1973.

12. Martin, M., Streptokinase stability pattern during storage in various solvents and at different temperatures, *Thrombos. Diathes. haemorrh. (Stuttg.)*, 33, 586, 1975.

13. Martin, M., Zur Kinetik der Aktivatorbildung unter fibrinolytischer Behandlung mit Streptokinase. Vortrag gehalten anläblich der 20, *Tagung Dtsch. Arbeitsgemeinschaft Blutgerinnungsforschung*, 2, 19, 1976.

14. Martin, M., Studies on activator formation in human plasma with streptokinase. III. Investigation of activator kinetics in undiluted plasma in terms of urokinase equivalents, *Thrombos. Haemostas. (Stuttgart)*, 1976.

15. Müllertz, S., Formation and properties of activator of plasminogen and of human and bovine plasmin, *Biochem. J.*, 61, 424, 1955.

16. Nachman, R. L., Immunologic studies of platelet protein, *Blood*, 25, 703, 1965.

17. Nussenzweig, V., Seligmann, M., Pelmont, J., and Grabar, P., Les produits de dégradation du fibrinogène humain par la plasmine. I - Séparation et propriétés physicochimiques, *Ann. Inst. Pasteur*, 100, 377, 1961.

18. DeRenzo, E. C., Chemistry of fibrinolysis (discussion), *Thrombos. Diathes. haemorrh. (Stuttg.)* Suppl. 1 and 6, 134, 1961.

19. Robbins, K. C., Bernabe, P., Arzadon, L., and Summaria, L., NH₂-terminal sequences of mammalian plasminogens and plasmin S-carboxymethyl heavy (A) and light (B) chain derivates, *J. Biol. Chem.*, 248, 7242, 1973.

20. Schwick, H. G., Biochemie der Fibrinolyse, in *Biologie des Plasmins; Purpura-Schönlein-Henoch, Erythrozytäre Gerinnungsaktivität*, Kunzer, W., Winckelmann, G., and Walter, Ch., Eds., F. K. Schattauer-Verlag, Stuttgart, 1967, 27.

21. Seligmann, M., and Marder, V., Application des techniques immunochimiques à l'étude du fibrinogène et de ses produits de dégradation par la plasmine, *Nouv. Rev. Fr. Hemat.*, 5, 345, 1965.

22. Summaria, L., Arzadon, L., Bernabe, P., and Robbins, K. C., The interaction of streptokinase with human, cat, dog and rabbit plasminogen, *J. Biol. Chem.*, 248, 4760, 1974.

23. Stachurska, J., Latallo, Z. S., and Kopec, M., Inhibition of platelet aggregation by dialysable fibrinogen degradation products (FDP), *Thrombos. Diathes. haemorrh. (Stuttg.)*, 23, 91, 1970.

24. Telesforo, P., Semeraro, N., Verstraete, M., and Collen, D., The inhibition of plasmin by antithrombin III - heparin complex in vitro in human plasma and during streptokinase therapy in man, *Thromb. Res.*, 7, 669, 1975.

25. Tillet, W. S. and Garner, R. L., The fibrinolytic activity of hemolytic streptococci, *J. Exp. Med.*, 58, 485, 1933.

Chapter 3

MECHANISMS OF THROMBOLYSIS INITIATED BY STREPTOKINASE

According to findings referred to in Chapter 2, Section V, activator formation process represents kinetic events characterized by the formula: streptokinase (SK) + plasminogen (Plg) $\rightleftharpoons$ activator (SK-Plg), and would seem to point to a reaction along the lines of the mass action law.

The clinical significance of the activator formation during streptokinase infusion is based on its ability to trigger the human plasminogen-plasmin conversion. According to figures provided by Schwick[1], a complete plaminogen-plasmin conversion comes into effect if 1/10 of the plasminogen molecules are bound to streptokinase for activator complex formation. The rest of the plasminogen molecules are converted to plasmin by action of the preformed activator. This course of events may be expressed by the schematic sequence of:

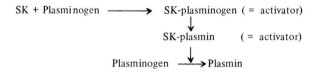

and can be referred to as "*inter*molecular plasminogen formation". However, as already mentioned, plasminogen, once trapped within the activator complex, readily converts to plasmin, the latter dissociating into the solvent medium. This kind of plasmin production may be called "*intra*molecular plasmin formation". It can be diagramed as follows:

$$
\begin{array}{l}
\text{SK + Plasminogen} \longrightarrow \text{SK-plasminogen (= activator)} \\
\qquad\qquad\qquad\qquad\qquad \downarrow \\
\qquad\qquad\qquad\quad \text{SK-plasmin} \qquad (= \text{activator}) \\
\qquad\qquad\qquad\quad \swarrow \qquad \searrow \\
\qquad\qquad\qquad \text{Plasmin} \quad \text{SK}
\end{array}
$$

No definite answer can be given yet to the question of clot dissolution mechanisms in vivo. From the theoretical point of view, three possibilities exist (Figure 1):

1. Streptokinase reacts with plasminogen, thus forming activator. Subsequently, by activator action plasmin is formed. Plasmin digests the external layer of the thrombus ("exogenous lysis").
2. Streptokinase reacts with plasminogen, thus forming activator. The activator penetrates the thrombus material. Plasmin appears in the thrombus interior by action of activator. Lysis starts in the inner parts of the thrombus ("endogenous lysis I").
3. Streptokinase penetrates thrombus material. Streptokinase reacts with plasminogen in the thrombus interior, thus forming activator. Activator converts plasminogen to plasmin. Lysis starts in the inner parts of the thrombus ("endogenous lysis II").

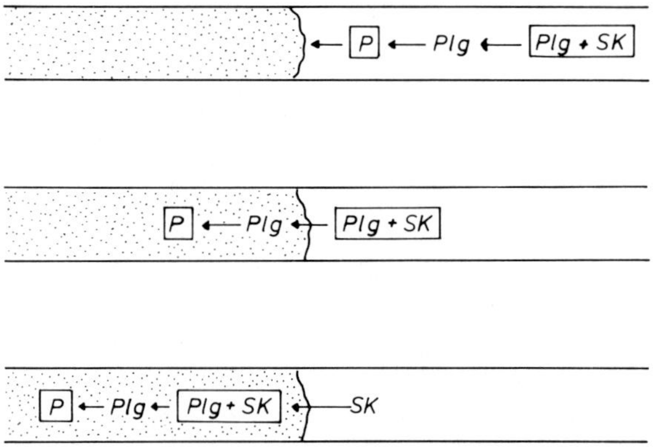

FIGURE 1.   Three possible thrombolytic mechanisms in vivo. Top: SK infused into the circulation is bound to plasminogen, thus forming the activator molecule. Activator acts on plasminogen, converting it to plasmin. Plasmin digests the superficial layers of the fibrin containing thrombus masses ("exogenous lysis"). Middle: Streptokinase reacts with plasminogen, thus forming activator. Activator invades thrombus material and converts plasminogen into plasmin. Lysis starts in the inner parts of the clot ("endogenous lysis I"). Bottom: Streptokinase invades thrombus material. In the gaps of the fibrin network, SK combines with plasminogen to activator. Activator converts plasminogen attached to the fibrin strands into plasmin. Lysis starts in the inner parts of the clot ("endogenous lysis II").

REFERENCE

1. **Schwick, H. G.,** Biochemie der Fibrinolyse, in *Biologie des Plasmin; Purpura-Schönlein-Henoch, Erythrozytäre Gerinnungsaktivität,* Kunzer, W., Winckelmann, G., and Walter, Ch., Eds., F. K. Schattauer-Verlag, Stuttgart, 1967, 27.

Chapter 4

BASIC GUIDELINES FOR STREPTOKINASE TREATMENT USING A SCHEMATIC DOSAGE REGIMEN*

All fibrinolytic procedures were carried out on patients who were required to remain in bed. However, the patient was allowed to get up for washing, for oscillographic measurement, and for bowel movements. This radius of activity was provided for by a 2 m infusion tube (Perfusor infusion set, B. Braun, Melsungen, West Germany) connecting the patient with the pump (Figure 1).

The single steps of the fibrinolytic procedures were as follows. A vein of the left distal forearm was punctured by inserting a plastic needle (Braunula No. 1/G 16, B. Braun, Melsungen, West Germany). Thereafter, a catheter (Intravascular Catheter for Braunula No. 1/G 16, B. Braun, Melsungen, West Germany) was eased into the plastic cannula. The catheter was shortened so as not to pass the elbow joint, and remained in place until termination of treatment. In case of phlebitis developing during infusion, the tip of the catheter was cut off thereby shortened by 2 to 3 cm. The infusion tube was connected with the syringe containing the streptokinase loading dose. After filling the infusion tube, its cone was fixed to the catheter's fitting. Great stress was laid on proper fixation of catheter and needle with adhesive tape. Subsequently, a second mandrin-closed Braunula needle (Stylet for Braunula No. 1/G 16, B. Braun, Melsungen, West Germany) was inserted into a vein of the right forearm in order to draw blood samples.

All infusions were carried out by an electric pump (Unita I, B. Braun, Melsungen, West Germany). Two Unita I glass syringes with metal plungers were filled with the exact amount of streptokinase** binding the circulating anti-SK content (CAC) or with a standard loading dose of 250,000 u streptokinase dissolved in 30 mℓ 5% glucose solution and 2.5 million u streptokinase dissolved in 50 mℓ 5% glucose solution, respectively.

Before starting therapy, a catalog of standardized items was checked:

1. Blood pressure
2. ECG for arrhythmia
3. History of cerebral disorders
4. Medication up to the day of treatment
5. Coagulation values (prothrombin time, partial thromboplastin time, fibrinogen, platelet count)

Patients under streptokinase treatment were examined every 2 hr around the clock. Forms were at hand for checking the following items three times per day:

1. Fever
2. Headache
3. Bleeding
4. Proper operation of infusion machine

---

* Some paragraphs in this chapter have been prepublished by M. Martin in *Progr. Cardiovasc. Dis.*, 21, 5, 1979. We thank Grune & Stratton for the permission to reprint these items.
** The streptokinase brand exclusively used in this study was Streptase®, Behringwerke AG, Marburg, Lahn, West Germany.

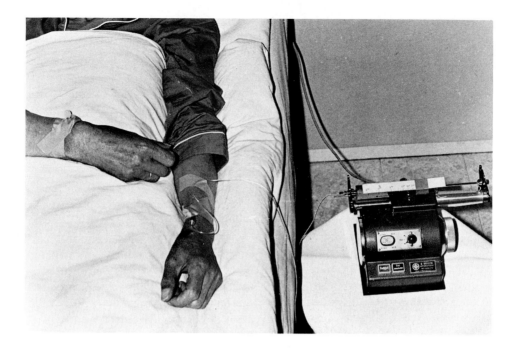

FIGURE 1.   Technical equipment for streptokinase treatment. Plastic cannulas (Braunulas) were inserted into the veins of both forearms. The right one was occluded by a stylet and destined for blood drawing. A catheter was introduced into the left one and connected with the infusion tube. The Unita I infusion machine was installed beside the bed. A time marker was fixed on the Unita I syringe (containing the streptokinase solution) for controlling the proper furtherance of the syringe plunger.

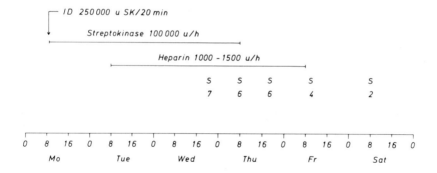

FIGURE 2.   Dosage scheme for schematic streptokinase-heparin treatment. Streptokinase, heparin, and acenocoumarol administrations overlap. In the schematic scheme the loading dose (ID) totaled 250,000 u/SK in every case, independent of the actual circulating anti-SK content (CAC).

Control of infusion machine was made possible by a time scale attached to the syringe. Proper operation was confirmed by agreement of plunger position and time shown on the scale.

Excitable patients were allowed such sedatives as diazepam (Valium 10, Hoffmann-LaRoche AG, Grenzach/Baden, West Germany). More effective soporifics, however, were not given on the grounds that the attending nurse, on her rounds, might be unable to make a proper assessment of the patient's well-being.

In order to neutralize the circulating anti-SK content of the patient (CAC), strepto-

Table 1
DISTRIBUTION OF EARLY
REACTION SIGNS

Flush	7%
Dyspnea	6%
Backache	15%
Flush + Dyspnea	10%
Flush + Backache	0%
Dyspnea + Backache	7%
Flush + Dyspnea + Backache	7%
	52%

Note: One or more of these reactions was found in
52% of the patients undergoing streptokinase
treatment.

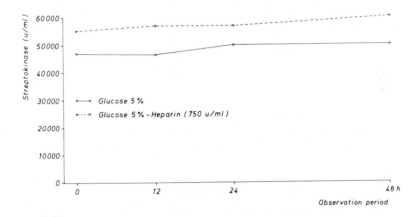

FIGURE 3. Stability pattern of 50,000 u/SK during storage in 1 mℓ each of 5% glucose and 5% glucose-750 u/mℓ heparin solution. There was no loss of streptokinase concentration over a period of 48 hr.

kinase treatment started with the infusion of a schematic loading dose (ID = initial dose) of 250,000 u SK (Figure 2). Since 90% of our patients displayed CACs below 250,000 anti-SK units (see Chapter 2, Section VII), this schematic procedure turned out to be fairly effective. The loading dose (250,000 u SK dissolved in 30 mℓ glucose solution) was infused with a speed of 90 mℓ/hr (position 9 on the Unita I scale) and completed after 20 min.

In about 50% of the patients, "early reactions", i.e., signs of flush, dyspnea, or backache, were recorded during the first 5 min of infusion (Table 1). In these cases the infusion was halted and 50 mg prednisolone injected. The patients were not unduly disturbed because they had been told in advance that the above symptoms were to be expected, that they were of short duration, and that they would not do any harm. The early reactions having subsided, the infusion of the loading dose was completed. Subsequently, the second syringe containing 2.5 million u SK/50 mℓ was put into the infusion machine. A new infusion tube was connected to the syringe, the tube was filled and then fixed on the patient's side at the catheter's fitting.

In order to arrive at the planned infusion rate of 100,000 u SK/hr, the pump had to be adjusted to a flow velocity of 2 mℓ/hr (position 10 on the Unita I scale). The infusion was supposed to run over a period of 25 hr without any change. Earlier investigation had proved that there was virtually no streptokinase concentration loss in a 2.5 million u SK/50 mℓ solution incubated for 48 hr at room temperature (Figure 3) (Martin[2]; Auel and Martin[1]).

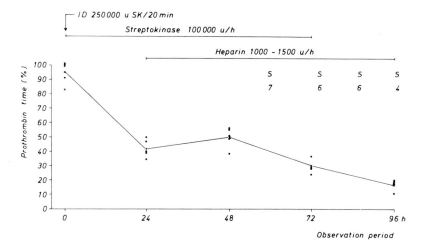

FIGURE 4.   Prothrombin times during a standardized streptokinase infusion series. Acenocoumarin (Sintrom®) medication was started 12 hr prior to ending SK infusion.

For the next 2 days a mixed streptokinase-heparin infusion was provided: 2.5 million u streptokinase and 37,500 u heparin were drawn up into the 50 mℓ Unita I syringe with 5% glucose solution, thus providing an infusion rate of both 100,000 u SK/hr and 1500 u heparin/hr (flow 2 mℓ/hr, position 10 on the Unita I scale).

Earlier studies have shown that heparin did not interfere with streptokinase stability in a streptokinase-heparin mixture (Martin[2]) (Figure 3).

At the beginning of the next day (third day of treatment) a PTT test was performed. PTT values between 50 and 90 sec were estimated as being in the therapeutic range. PTT values above 90 sec warranted a reduction of the heparin inflow down to 1000 u/hr. PTT values below the 50 sec mark (i.e., nearly normal values) led to an elevation of the heparin inflow to 2000 u/hr.

Half a day before terminating the streptokinase-heparin infusion, an additional acenocoumarol (Sintrom®) treatment was started (28 mg in the evening, 48 mg next day, 16 mg on following day). Under this coumarol regimen a prothrombin time within the therapeutic range was normally reached after 2 ½ days medication (Figure 4). The drawing of blood samples for prothrombin time determination was always carried out after the infusion machine had been turned off for at least 2 hr.

After the streptokinase infusion was stopped, heparin ran alone until the prothrombin time had arrived at therapeutic levels of between 15 to 25% (recording of the prothrombin value 2 hr after turning off the heparin inflow).

Having removed the infusion equipment on the left arm and the blood-drawing needle on the right arm, a tight elastic dressing was laid to avoid puncture wound bleeding. The dressing was removed 2 days later.

REFERENCES

1. **Auel, H. and Martin, M.,** Die Technik des quantitativen Streptokinasenachweises im Plasma, *Klin. Wochenschr.,* 53, 809, 1975.
2. **Martin, M.,** Streptokinase stability pattern during storage in various solvents and at different temperatures, *Thrombos. Diathes. Haemorrh. (Stuttg.),* 33, 586, 1975.

Chapter 5

CONTRAINDICATION FOR STREPTOKINASE TREATMENT*

Contraindications should be ruled out before a patient is admitted to fibrinolytic treatment. Contraindications mandatory for streptokinase therapy include:

1. Gastric ulcer
2. Hypertension (i.e., diastolic pressure above 100 mmHg)
3. History of cerebral accidents (stroke, hemorrhage, severe newly developing headache, history of severe cerebral trauma, etc.)
4. General bleeding disorders
5. Major surgery within the last 4 days
6. Confinement within the last 4 weeks
7. Cancer, leukemia

Optional contraindications are

1. Age above 65 years
2. I.M. injections within the last 2 weeks
3. Liver diseases
4. Renal failure
5. Atrial fibrillation
6. Earlier streptokinase therapy — 3 days to 3 months previously
7. Menorrhagia
8. Intake of anticoagulants or thrombocyte-active drugs

Hypertension being established, pretreatment with antihypertensive drugs such as Clonidine (Catapresan, C. H. Boehringer Sohn, Ingelheim, West Germany) might normalize the blood pressure and enable the physician to perform streptokinase treatment 3 or 4 days later.

A cerebral accident under lytic treatment has to be looked upon as the most dangerous side effect involved. A scrupulous history and neurologic examination with rejection of patients showing any signs of cerebral alterations is called for.

Since a period of reduced resistance against commonplace infections (flu, angina, bronchitis, etc.) was occasionally observed after streptokinase treatment, **a frail constitution,** as seen in elderly patients beyond 65 to 70 years of age, might be regarded as an optional contraindication for lytic treatment.

Intramuscular injection administered less than 14 days before streptokinase treatment includes the risk of muscular bleeding (see Chapter 14). Because of unbearable pain, muscular bleeding inevitably led to termination of treatment.

Streptokinase might be metabolized in the liver[6] and the derivatives excreted with the urine.[1] Therefore, **liver diseases and renal failure** must be taken into account. Plasma streptokinase checks (Chapter 16, Section VI) during treatment are then advisable.

Atrial fibrillation on the basis of mitral stenosis and/or left atrial dilation might lead to thrombus formation in the left atrium. Arterial embolization (into the cerebrum, among other localities) can be induced by lytic treatment. Mitral stenosis with

---

* Some paragraphs in this chapter have been prepublished by M. Martin in *Prog. Cardiovasc. Dis.,* 21, 5, 1979. We thank Grune & Stratton for the permission to reprint these items.

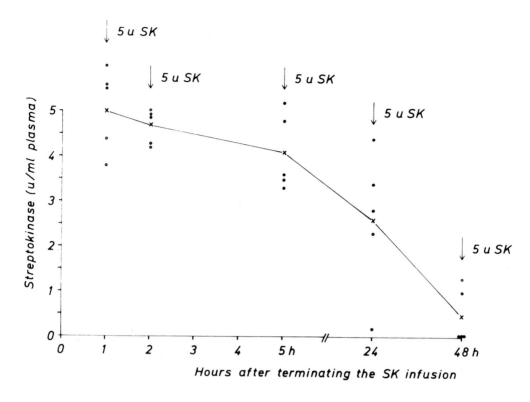

FIGURE 1.   Demonstration of rising antistreptokinase titers after streptokinase treatment. 5 u SK were transferred into 1 mℓ plasma aliquots obtained from patients 1, 2, 5, 24 and 48 hr after terminating SK infusion. As can be seen from the chart, nearly all of the streptokinase units transferred into the post-lysis plasma were recovered during the first 4 hr. By contrast, a considerable loss of streptokinase was recorded 24 hr and 48 hr after terminating SK infusion, thus indicating a subsequent rise in anti-SK activity.

atrial fibrillation can, therefore, be regarded as optional contraindication for lytic therapy. By contrast, patients with longstanding atrial fibrillation due to coronary heart disease were frequently SK-treated without any signs of embolization. According to our experience, the coronary type of atrial fibrillation should not be included in the contraindication table.

A second series of streptokinase treatment is an optional contraindication if the time interval between the two series is longer than 3 days and less than 3 months. Immediately after ending streptokinase treatment, the anti-SK titer is virtually zero. Antibody production starts very slowly and reaches the 5 anti-SK units/mℓ* after about 2 days[5] (Figure 1). The highest peak of anti-SK content, climbing to values around 30 million, was found 2 ½ weeks after cessation of treatment. A decline to normal or subnormal values was found after 3 months.[2] However, even if anti-SK values are low during the first week after streptokinase treatment, a booster effect can be induced by the second effort of lytic therapy (Figure 2). Conceivably, such a powerful rise in anti-SK cannot be overcome by a conventional streptokinase regimen.

CAC-values above 1 million anti-SK units without a previous history of streptokinase treatment are by no means contraindications for lytic treatment. According to our experience, lysis starts regularly once the amount of titrated CAC is infused (see Chapter 7, Section II). However, the inflow procedures should be monitored closely. After influx of a first 50,000 u SK amount, a 4 min pause should be made. Following

* Equalling a circulating antibody content of about 12,500 anti-SK u.

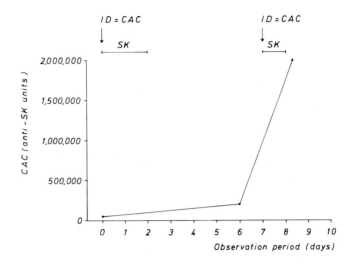

FIGURE 2. Booster effect on anti-SK production in a patient who received two SK infusion series with an interval of 5 days between them. The second treatment series was terminated because of absent lytic effects (no decrease in fibrinogen, no prolongation of PTT).

the second 50,000 u SK, a 4 min pause should be made. Following the second 50,000 u SK, a 4 min pause should be made. Following the second 50,000 u SK, another 4 min pause is recommended. After that, the regular schedule may be carried out. If the above precautions are taken, the incidence rate of early reactions is not higher than in patients with low CAC values. For handling early reactions, see Chapter 4.

Menstrual bleeding does not raise major problems under lytic treatment. However, in case of menorrhagia, streptokinase therapy should possibly be avoided. Menstrual bleeding expected within the next couple of days can be postponed by administering 2 mg 17α-ethinyl-19-nortestosterone acetate + 0.01 mg ethinylestradiol (Primosiston-Tbl., Schering AG, West Berlin) t.i.d. According to Ludwig[4] streptokinase treatment can be carried out during pregnancy from the 14th week onward. Since neither streptokinase nor heparin penetrate the placental barrier,[7] streptokinase treatment seems possible during pregnancy from the 15th week onward.[4] Furthermore, streptokinase therapy may be performed 4 to 5 days after delivery. In order to avoid genital bleeding, an additional treatment with oxytoxic agents (Oxytocin, 3 u I.V. t.i.d.) may be necessary.

Patients on oral anticoagulants with prothrombin times well below 20% were pretreated with Vitamin K₁ (Phytomenadion, Konakion®, Hoffmann-LaRoche AG, Grenzach/Baden, West Germany) 1 mg I.V. Subsequently, streptokinase treatment started under prothrombin values above 25%.

In order to avoid bleeding tendencies, intake of **antiadhesive drugs,** such as acetylsalicylic acid (Aspirin, Colfarit, Bayer AG, Leverkusen, West Germany), should be stopped several days before lysis is planned.

REFERENCES

1. **Fletcher, A. P., Alkjaersig, N., and Sherry, S.,** The clearance of heterologous protein from the circulation of normal and immunized man, *J. Clin. Invest.,* 37, 1306, 1958.
2. **Köstering, H., Barth, U. and Naidu, R.,** Changes in antistreptokinase titers following long term streptokinase therapy, in *New Concepts in Streptokinase Dosimetry,* Hans Huber, Bern, 1978.
3. **Ludwig, H.,** Thrombolytic therapy in pregnancy. Experimental and clinical studies, *Thrombos. Diathes. Haemorrh. (Stuttg.),* 47, (Suppl.) 243, 1971.
4. **Ludwig, H.,** Results of streptokinase therapy in deep venous thrombosis during pregnancy, *Postgrad. Med. J.,* 5, (Suppl.), 65, 1973.
5. **Martin, M.,** Indirect measurement of streptokinase concentration in the plasma of patients undergoing fibrinolytic treatment, *Thrombos. Diathes. haemorrh. (Stuttg.),* 32, 633, 1974.
6. **Pfeiffer, G. W.,** Zur Pharmakokinetik von 131 J-Streptokinase am Menschen, *Klin. Wochenschr.,* 47, 482, 1969.
7. **Pfeiffer, G. W.,** The use of thrombolytic therapy in obstetrics and gynecology, *Aust. Ann. Med.,* 19 (Suppl. 1), 28, 1970.

Chapter 6

CLINICAL METHODS FOR CONTROLLING BLOOD VESSEL PATENCY

In the course of lytic treatment of arterial occlusions as surveyed in this study, an angiogram was at hand in 90% of the cases prior to, and in 40% after streptokinase infusion. In the group of "successfully treated" occlusions, angiography was present in 82% of the cases before, and in 48% after treatment.

Arterial stenoses were checked angiographically prior to treatment in 93% of the cases, and rechecked after termination of treatment in 44%.

Reasons for not carrying out angiography prior to streptokinase infusion were based mainly on the time factor. Being briefed that lytic success in thrombosed arteries decreases rapidly after an occlusion period of 2 weeks, we felt that, in a number of patients, no time was left for angiographic procedures and puncture wound healing. In these cases, the diagnosis was proved only by clinical methods (see below), and streptokinase infusion started without delay. Likewise, in a certain number of instances, recheck angiograms could not be carried out because the respective patient, having regained a walking distance of unlimited length, would decline to undergo further invasive diagnostic procedures.

Before treating *arterial stenoses,* an angiogram was generally in existence (93%). This was regarded as mandatory because the indication for lytic treatment depended, *inter alia,* on the morphological structure of the narrowing (see Chapter 10). Angiographic rechecks, on the other hand, were often abstained from because of their non-reliability for proving a hemodynamically significant widening.[6] Here, clinical methods, such as ultrasonic pressure measurements, seemed of much greater relevance.

Clinical methods for evaluating vessel patency consisted of:

- Pulse palpation
- Auscultation
- Oscillometry at rest
- Oscillometry after exercise
- Ultrasonic Doppler pressure measurements

All oscillometry measurements were performed with the mechanical oscillograph of Gesenius and Keller (Speidel & Keller K.G., Jungingen, West Germany). In this device, air-filled cuffs for pressure conduction and Murray's capsule as pressure sensor are used. Thigh, calf, and ankle oscillography at rest, as well as ankle oscillometry following standardized heel-raising and knee-bending exercises[2,7] were regularly performed.

Bilateral oscillometry *at rest* was carried out by stepwise pressure reduction from 160 to 40 mmHg. Oscillometry *after exercise* included heel-raising 40 times and knee-bends 20 times. During and after exercise oscillometry, cuffs were placed above the ankles. Exactly 15 sec after terminating exercises, oscillometric curves were recorded. Normally, no reduction in oscillometric amplitudes occurred after exercise. However, stenoses and/or occlusions present in aortic, iliac, femoral, and popliteal vessels led to a considerable reduction in the magnitude of oscillations for a variable period of time, the latter being dependent on the grade of hemodynamic impediment involved.

Ultrasonic pressure measurements were performed according to Franklin et al.[3], Bollinger et al., Schoop and Levy[8], Martin[4], and Martin et al.[5] In the latter method, cuffs were placed around the ankles and inflated up to 300 mmHg. Subsequently, the pressure was reduced until first flow signals were recorded in the posterior tibial artery by means of ultrasonic Doppler technique. This pressure figure was referred to as "systolic ankle pressure". In order to calculate the systolic pressure gradient along the occlusion, the systolic blood pressure (systemic pressure) on the upper arm was measured and the ankle pressure subtracted.

As an example, the following data accumulated from a patient undergoing fibrinolytic treatment are presented:

Before Treatment
- Pulse Palpation

Inguinal pulse	right +	left +
Popliteal pulse	right 0	left +
Posterior tibial artery	right 0	left +
Anterior tibial artery	right 0	left +

- Auscultation
  No bruits along the iliac, femoral, and popliteal arteries

- Oscillometry at Rest
  Right side: reduction of ankle amplitudes
  Left side: normal oscillations

- Oscillometry After Exercise
  Right side: after heel-raising and knee-bends, disappearance of oscillations for 4 min
  Left side: normal oscillations after heel-raising and knee-bends

- Ultrasonic Doppler Pressure Measurement

Upper arm (systemic pressure)	140 mmHg
Right ankle (tib. post. a.)	35 mmHg
Left ankle (tib. post. a.)	150 mmHg

The clinical diagnosis drawn from the above data was "femoral occlusion on the right side".

After Treatment
- Pulse Palpation

Inguinal pulse	right +	left +
Popliteal pulse	right +	left +
Posterior tibial artery	right +	left +
Anterior tibial artery	right +	left +

- Auscultation
  Systolic bruit along the medium part of the right femoral artery. Left: no bruits

- Oscillometry at Rest
  Right side: normal oscillation
  Left side: normal oscillation

- Oscillometry After Exercise
  Right side: normal oscillations after both heel-raising and knee-bends
  Left side: normal oscillations after both heel-raising and knee-bends

- Ultrasonic Doppler Pressure Measurement
  Upper arm (systemic pressure)   130 mmHg

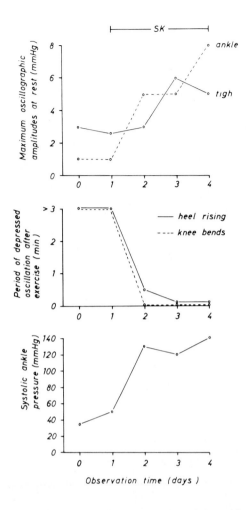

FIGURE 1. Synoptic representation of the results of oscillometry at rest and after exercise, as well as of ankle pressure measurements in a patient on whom a lytic treatment was conducted and where a femoral occlusion was removed on the second day of streptokinase therapy.

Right ankle (tib. post. a.)   140 mmHg
Left ankle (tib. post. a.)   140 mmHg

The conclusions drawn from the above data were "removal of a right femoral artery occlusion by lytic treatment; residue of a stenosis without major effect". A schematic representation of this sequence of events is given in Figure 1.

The respective pre- and post-treatment angiograms are shown in Figure A-3 of the Appendix.

In some cases, the clinical assessment would have led to a false negative conclusion if angiography had not been carried out. For example, one patient, displaying a common iliac occlusion, a severely narrowed external iliac artery and a femoral occlusion, was treated by streptokinase. The therapeutic effects seemed to be negative (no definite changes in pulse palpation, auscultation, oscillography). Yet, the recheck angiogram showed total clearance of the common iliac segment while the external iliac stenosis and the femoral occlusion were still in existence (see Appendix, Figure A-6).

REFERENCES

1. **Bollinger, A., Mahler, F., and Zehender, O.**, Kombinierte Druck- und Durchflubmessungen in der Beurteilung arterieller Durchblutungsstörungen, *Dtsch. Med. Wochenschr.,* 95, 1039, 1970.
2. **Ejrup, B.,** Tonoscillographie after exercise, *Acta Med. Scand.,* 5, (Suppl.), 285, 1948.
3. **Franklin, D. L., Schlegel, W., and Rushmer, R. F.**, Blood flow measured by Doppler frequency shift of back scattered ultrasound, *Science,* 134, 564, 1961.
4. **Martin, M.**, Ultrasonic Doppler measurement of systolic pressure in the quantitative evaluation of chronic arterial occlusions, *J. Am. Geriatr. Soc.,* 28, 349, 1980.
5. **Martin, M., Müller-Scholtes, G. M., and Auel, H.**, Die systolische Blutdruckmessung mit Hilfe der Ultraschall-Doppler-Technik bei Gesunden und VerschluBkranken *VASA,* 8, 4, 1979.
6. **Martin, M., Schoop, W., and Zeitler, E.**, Thrombolyse bei chronischer Arteriopathie, *Verl. Hans Huber,* Bern, 1970.
7. **Schoop, W. and Lehner, M.**, Belastungsoszillographie mit dem Apparat nach Gesenius-Keller, *Med. Welt,* 35, 1721, 1963.
8. **Schoop, W. and Levy, H.**, Messung des systolischen Blutdruckes distal eines Extremitätenverschlusses mit Hilfe der Ultraschall-Doppler-Technik, *Verh. Dtsch. Ges. Kreisl.-Forsch.,* 35, 456, 1969.

Chapter 7

LABORATORY DATA COLLECTED DURING STREPTOKINASE INFUSION*

I. GENERAL REMARKS ON SKAPPFF DETERMINATION (STREPTOKINASE, ACTIVATOR, PLASMINOGEN, PLASMIN, FIBRINOGEN, AND FDP MEASUREMENTS)

The exact state of fibrinolytic activities present in the plasma of patients under streptokinase infusion might be best characterized by the simultaneous recording of:

- Streptokinase concentration
- Activator concentration
- Plasminogen concentration
- Plasmin concentration
- Fibrinogen concentration
- Fibrinogen degradation products (FDP)

The following paragraphs deal with SKAPPFF profiles derived from various forms of streptokinase treatment. Streptokinase (u/mℓ plasma), activator (urokinase equivalent, CTA-u/mℓ plasma), and plasminogen concentrations (% of normal) were measured according to Martin.[14-16] Plasmin (expressed in novo u/mℓ plasma) was measured on heated bovine fibrin plates according to Lassen[12], modified by Martin[15]. For further methodic details, see Chapter 16.

II. LABORATORY DATA COLLECTED DURING STREPTOKINASE TREATMENT STARTED BY A STREPTOKINASE INITIAL DOSE (ID) EQUALING THE TOTAL AMOUNT OF CIRCULATING ANTI-SK CONTENT (CAC) (= SK REGIMEN A)

SKAPPFF measurements were carried out in 12 patients. Before treatment, CACs were determined. The following values were recorded:

Patient's Ref. No.	CAC
584	63,500
585	147,000
591	31,000
596	241,500
598	252,000
604	112,000
605	13,000
607	43,000
609	30,000
612	89,000
619	480,000
620	1,057,000

---

* Some paragraphs in this chapter have been prepublished by M. Martin in *Prog. Cardiovasc. Dis.*, 21, 5, 1979. We thank Grune & Stratton for the permission to reprint these items.

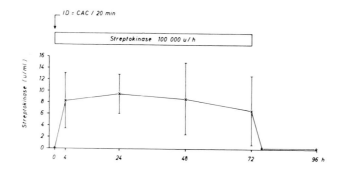

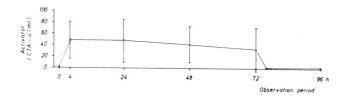

FIGURE 1.   Streptokinase and activator concentations in 11 patients during the course of SK dosage regimen A (ID = CAC, MD = 100,000 u SK/hr).

Obviously, a wide spectrum of CACs from 13,000 to 1,057,000 anti-SK u resulted. The SK inflow scheme consisted of administering a loading dose equaling the exact amount of CAC over a period of 20 min. After that, a maintenance dose (MD) of 100,000 u SK/hr was administered up to the 75th hr of treatment.

SKAPPFF measurements were performed before treatment (0) and 4 hr, 24 hr, 48 hr, 72 hr, and 96 hr after starting the 3 day infusion series.

Between the 4th and 72nd hr of treatment, the following SKAPPFF characteristics were recorded. *Streptokinase* concentration was recorded at between 8 and 10 u/ml during the first 2 days of treatment, falling to 6 u/ml thereafter (Figure 1). *Activator concentrations* ran steadily around 40 CTA u/ml (Figure 1). During the first 4 hr of streptokinase infusion, plasminogen went straight down to below 1% and was afterwards found around 0.5%, with only minor changes during the whole infusion period. After terminating streptokinase infusion, plasminogen recovered rather quickly and reached the 50% mark after a period of 24 hr (Figure 2). No *plasmin* was traceable between the 4th and 72nd hr of infusion.

The lowest *fibrinogen* concentration was measured 24 hr after starting treatment. It fell from an initial 420 mg% to 150 mg%. After that, despite further streptokinase infusion, a steady rise to values of 200 mg% was observed. The fibrinogen level had reached 250 mg% 24 hr after cessation of treatment (Figure 3).

Coagulation active *fibrinogen degradation products* (FDP), expressed in terms of corrected reptilase time (cRT), were only found to be elevated 4 hr after start of treatment. Thereafter (24 hr, 48 hr, 72 hr, 96 hr) normal values were recorded (Figure 3).

Attention should be drawn to the fact that despite large differences in CAC values, the respective standard deviations of streptokinase, activator, plasminogen, fibrinogen and cRT values were relatively small. For example, 24 hr after starting streptokinase infusion, the means and standard deviations were as follows:

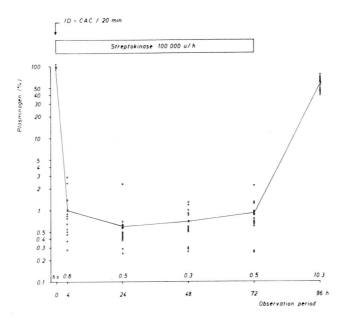

FIGURE 2.   Plasminogen concentrations in 12 patients during the course of SK dosage regimen A (ID = CAC, MD = 100,000 u SK/hr).

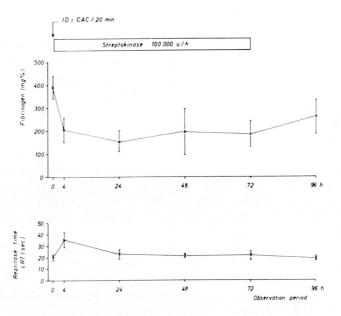

FIGURE 3.   Fibrinogen concentrations (gravimetric) and FDP activity in 12 patients during the course of SK dosage regimen A (ID = CAC, MD = 100,000 u SK/hr).

SK	9.5 ± 3.4 u/ml
Activator	48 ± 37.0 CTA u/ml
Plasminogen	0.6 ± 0.5%
Fibrinogen	196 ± 101 mg%
cRT	23 ± 4 sec

These figures indicate convincingly that the above streptokinase regimen (CAC = ID, MD = 100,000 u/hr) can be looked upon as a highly appropriate scheme for guaranteeing a uniform pattern of fibrinolytic reactions.

III. LABORATORY DATA COLLECTED DURING STREPTOKINASE TREATMENT STARTED AND MAINTAINED BY A SCHEMATIC DOSAGE REGIMEN (= SK REGIMEN B)

SKAPPFF measurements were carried out in six patients. Before treatment, CAC was determined. The following values were recorded:

Patient's ref. no.	CAC
413	33,000
415	33,000
416	122,000
417	231,000
419	28,000
426	24,000

According to these data, the CAC spectrum included values between 24,000 and 231,000 anti-SK units. As in the foregoing section, SKAPPFF determinations were carried out before treatment (0), during therapy (4 hr, 24 hr, 48 hr, 72 hr) and 24 hr after termination of treatment (96 hr).

The streptokinase infusion regimen consisted of administering a schematic loading dose of ID = 250,000 u SK/ 20 min, independent of the individual CAC measured. Subsequently, a maintenance dose of MD = 100,000 u SK/hr was infused over a period of 72 hr.

Streptokinase concentrations were averaging 8 u/ml plasma 4 hr after starting treatment. Thereafter, a constant decline in streptokinase concentration to 4 u/ml at the 72nd hr of treatment was observed (Figure 4).

The run of *activator* concentration movements were very similar to that of streptokinase. There was a peak of 120 CTA-u/ml after 4 hr of treatment, and a steady decline to 40 CTA-u/ml thereafter (Figure 4).

After 4 hr of treatment, *plasminogen* concentration fell to 0.85%. Later on, concentrations of between 0.5 and 0.1% were monitored but 24 hr after terminating treatment, plasminogen concentration again reached a value of 60% (Figure 5).

Plasmin was absent between the 4th and 72nd hr of streptokinase infusion.

Fibrinogen had its major drop during the first 24 hr, from an initial average value of 420 mg% to 162 mg%. Later on it recovered to values of 190 mg% after 72 hr (last hour of treatment), and 294 mg% (24 hr after ending SK infusion, i.e., 96th observation hour). (Figure 6).

The corrected reptilase time (cRT), as an indicator of circulating *fibrinogen degradation products* (FDP), was significantly prolonged only during the first 24 hr. Later on, normal or subnormal values were recorded (Figure 6).

The above data, accumulated in the course of SK regimen B (i.e., schematic loading dose of 250,000 u/SK) are of interest with respect to the clinical impact involved. Can both regimens — CAC-adapted form (SK regimen A) and CAC-independent form (SK

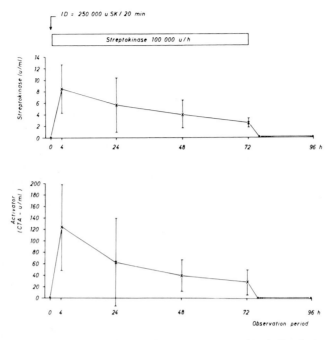

FIGURE 4.   Streptokinase and activator concentrations in 7 patients during the course of SK regimen B (CAC-independent scheme).

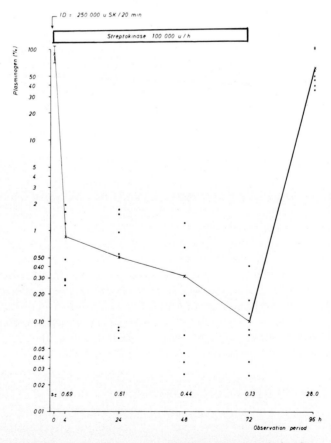

FIGURE 5.   Plasminogen concentrations in 7 patients during the course of SK regimen B (CAC-independent scheme).

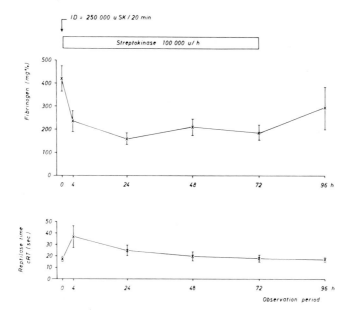

FIGURE 6.   Fibrinogen concentrations (gravimetric) and FDP activities (expressed in terms of cRT = fibrinogen-corrected reptilase time) in 7 patients during the course of SK regimen B (CAC-independent scheme).

regimen B) — be regarded equally suited for therapeutic purposes? To elucidate this problem, the average values of streptokinase activator, plasminogen, fibrinogen and FDP concentrations, together with their respective standard deviations, were compared in both groups 24 hr after starting treatment.

	SK Regimen A	SK Regimen B
SK	9.5 ± 3.4 u/ml	5.7 ± 4.7 u/ml
Activator	48 ± 37.0 CTA-u/ml	62.5 ± 77 CTA-u/ml
Plasminogen	0.6 ± 0.5%	0.51 ± 0.61%
Fibrinogen	196 ± 101 mg%	162 ± 25 mg%
cRT	23 ± 4 sec	25 ± 4.5 sec

As can be seen in the table, the average values and their respective standard deviations were virtually equal.

Abnormally high CAC values can, however, suppress lytic reactions for a considerable period of time. For example, one patient, displaying a CAC value of 2.45 million anti-SK u, underwent SK treatment according to SK regimen B (i.e., loading dose 250,000 u SK/20 min, maintenance dose 100,000 u SK/hr). In this case, streptokinase activity was not recorded until the 24th infusion hour (Figure 7), thereby wasting valuable time. However, keeping in mind that CAC values larger than 250,000 anti-SK u are below 10% in today's population (see Chapter 2), SK regimen B might be preferred to regimen A in emergency cases where no time is left for laboratory tests, and in facilities not equipped for performing the CAC measurements.

IV. LABORATORY DATA COLLECTED IN THE COURSE OF A SMALL DOSE REGIMEN (30,000 u SK/HR) (= SK REGIMEN C)

Several centers have provided evidence that fibrinolytic effects can be achieved by applying small dose streptokinase regimens, the maintenance dose (MD) being smaller than 100,000 u SK/hr.[3,5,7,8,10,13,19]

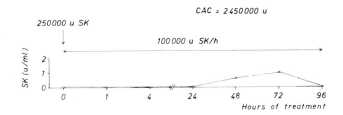

FIGURE 7.   Streptokinase concentration in the plasma of a patient
displaying a circulating anti-SK content (CAC) of 2.4 million prior to
treatment. First measurable SK quantities were not seen before the
24th hr of treatment.

In the following section SKAPPFF determinations, accumulated in the course of a
small dose regimen, are presented. The therapeutic scheme consisted of a loading dose
equaling the CAC, and a maintenance dose amounting to 30,000 u SK/hr.

In the respective patients, the following CAC values were recorded:

Patient's ref. no.	CAC
538	66,000
539	24,000
543	67,000
545	60,000
546	67,000
564	48,000
565	29,000
566	276,000
572	32,000
573	31,000

Streptokinase concentrations averaged 1 u/ml plasma throughout treatment (Figure
8).

Activator concentrations were concomitantly measurable, with values around 20
CTA-u/ml (Figure 8).

Interestingly, and in contrast to the regimens presented in the two foregoing chapters, the mean *plasminogen* concentration was running clearly above the 1% borderline
(Figure 9).

Another new feature in the sequence of the small dose streptokinase regimen was
the observation of a continuous *plasminemia* throughout treatment, averaging 0.015
novo u/ml (Figure 9). Surprisingly, this overt plasminemia did not lead to a *fibrinogen*
fall greater than that seen in the SK regimens A or B, in which much higher SK maintenance doses were applied and in which no plasminemia could be spotted (Figure 10).
After 24 hr SK small dose infusion, the fibrinogen concentration fell from an initial
360 mg% to 100 mg%. After that, a rise to 200 mg% was observed at the 24th and
72nd hr of treatment, respectively.

V. LABORATORY DATA COLLECTED IN THE COURSE OF A MINIDOSAGE REGIMEN (5000 u SK/HR) (= SK REGIMEN D)

In 1974, Dotter et al.[2] were able to show that arterial occlusions of thrombotic origin
could be removed by inserting a catheter into the thrombus material, with subsequent
infusion of 5000 u SK/hr via the catheter. Thus stimulated, our group has investigated
streptokinase activator, plasminogen, plasmin and fibrinogen concentrations under the
influence of this minidosage regimen.

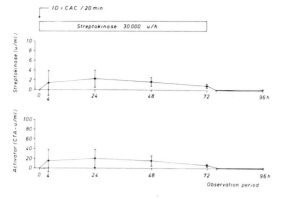

FIGURE 8.   Streptokinase and activator concentrations in
10 patients during the course of SK regimen C (small dose
regimen).

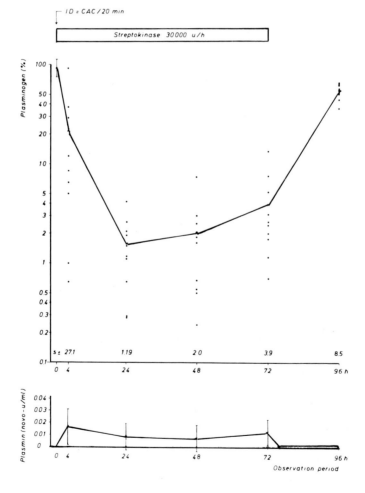

FIGURE 9.   Plasminogen and plasmin concentrations in 10 patients
during the course of SK regimen C (small dose regimen).

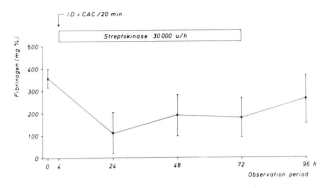

FIGURE 10. Fibrinogen concentrations (Schulz method) in 10 patients during the course of SK regimen C (small dose regimen).

CAC values in five patients tested so far were

Patient's ref. no.	CAC
487	340,000
488	128,000
489	48,000
495	23,000
497	1,245,000

During the first 20 min the exact CAC amount was infused. Subsequently, 5000 u/hr were administered over the next 24 hr.

As can be seen on the charts of Figures 11 and 12, *plasminogen* fell by 50%, *plasmin* was hardly recognizable, and there was only a very slight decrease in *fibrinogen*. *Streptokinase* and *activator* were not measurable by the assays applied in this study.

VI. LABORATORY DATA COLLECTED IN THE COURSE OF INTERMITTENT STREPTOKINASE ADMINISTRATION (= SK REGIMEN E)

Introducing an intermittent streptokinase dosage regimen adds a new and possibly advantageous aspect to the fibrinolytic treatment procedure. Intermittent treatment leads to additional periods of plasminemia at the beginning and the end of each streptokinase infusion series (see Sections IX and X). Furthermore, the streptokinase-induced plasminogen depletion is interrupted several times during the SK-free periods, thus providing reiteration of plasminogen penetration of thrombus material. Both elements might enhance intravascular clot dissolution.

Fibrinolytic parameters were studied in four patients displaying the following CAC values:

Patient's ref. no.	CAC
225	246,000
235	155,000
251	124,000
258	393,000

Treatment started by administering a loading dose, equaling the individual CAC, over 20 min. Subsequently, a maintenance dose of 100,000 u SK/hr was infused for

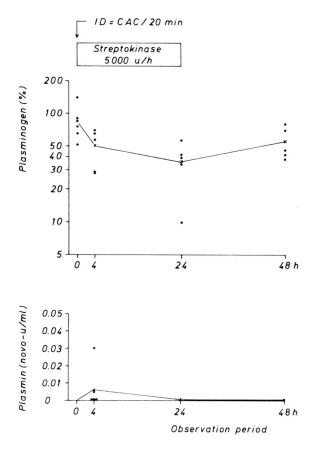

FIGURE 11.   Plasminogen and plasmin concentrations in 5 patients during the course of SK regimen D (minidosage).

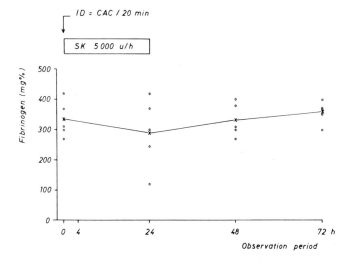

FIGURE 12.   Fibrinogen concentrations (Schulz method) in 5 patients during the course of SK regimen D (minidosage).

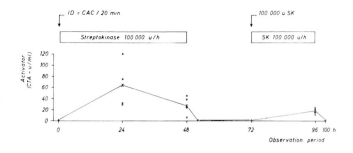

FIGURE 13. Activator concentrations in 4 patients during the course of intermittent streptokinase treatment.

24 hr. This was followed by a streptokinase-free interval of another 24 hr. The second streptokinase series started with a uniform initial dose of 100,000 u SK/5 min and went on with 100,000 u SK/hr over the next 24 hr.

During the intermittent streptokinase treatment, two peaks of *activator* concentration were recorded. In the first streptokinase series, an activator concentration of 60 CTA-u/ml at the 24th hr, and a much lower value of 24 CTA-u/ml at the 48th hr, were monitored. A relatively small peak of 18 CTA-u/ml was measured 24 hr after starting the second series. Conceivably, no activator activity appeared between the two SK infusion periods (Figure 13).

Plasminogen and activator concentrations acted in a reciprocal manner, i.e., an activator increase corresponded to a plasminogen drop, and an activator decrease to a plasminogen rise. Plasminogen fell below 0.5% during the first 4 hr and stayed there for the next 44 hr. Between the two infusion series, plasminogen rose to 50% and dropped again to below 0.5% upon administering the second SK infusion (Figure 14).

Fibrinogen concentrations ran in a sinusoidal shape, i.e., a first drop from 400 mg% to 150 mg% occurred during the first streptokinase infusion series, a rise from 150 mg% to 370 mg% was seen in the SK-free interval, and another drop from 370 mg% to 125 mg% took place during the second streptokinase administration period (Figure 15).

VII. LABORATORY DATA COLLECTED DURING TREATMENT WITH ESCALATING STREPTOKINASE INFLOW RATES (= SK REGIMEN F)

Five patients were infused daily with increasing amounts of streptokinase: 100,000 u/hr on the 1st day, 150,000 u/hr on the 2nd day, and 200,000 u/hr on the 3rd day of treatment. In each case the loading dose equaled the CAC value and was administered during the first 20 min. The CAC distribution was as follows:

Patient's ref. no.	CAC
515	280,000
516	574,000
518	56,000
523	69,000
524	32,000

After a 24 hr inflow of 100,000 u SK/hr, the *streptokinase* concentration averaged 10 u/ml. During the next 24 hr an infusion of 150,000 u/hr was administered, leading to a streptokinase concentration of 16 u/ml. This value was held despite another increase of the streptokinase infusion rate to 200,000 u/hr (Figure 16).

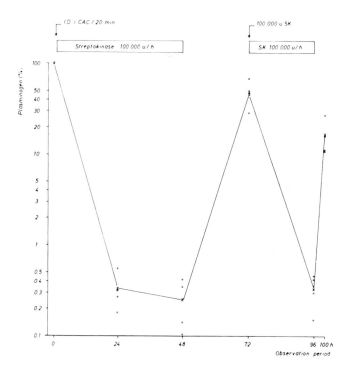

FIGURE 14.   Plasminogen concentrations in 4 patients during the course of intermittent streptokinase treatment.

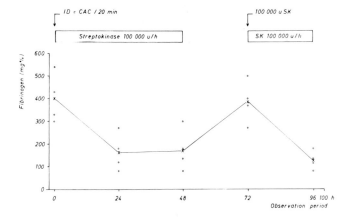

FIGURE 15.   Fibrinogen concentrations (Schulz method) in 4 patients during the course of intermittent streptokinase treatment.

The *activator* concentration values reacted in a similar pattern. After a continuous activator rise to 110 CTA-u/mℓ over the first 48 hr, the activator strength leveled off and stayed at 100 CTA-u/mℓ in spite of a further rise in streptokinase inflow (Figure 16).

During the whole course of the escalating streptokinase inflow regimen, *plasminogen* remained stable at concentrations of 0.2 to 0.3%. These values are similar to those seen in the customary 3 day streptokinase regimens of 100,000 u SK/hr. Obviously, streptokinase inflow rates above 100,000 u/hr do not lower the plasminogen level be-

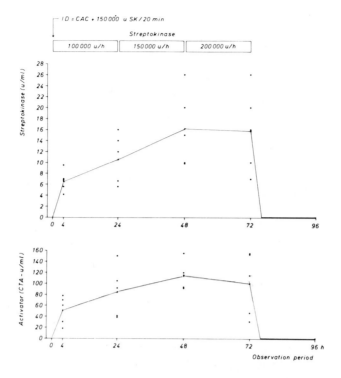

FIGURE 16. Streptokinase and activator concentrations in 5 patients under escalating SK inflow rates (1st day 100,000 u/hr, 2nd day 150,000 u/hr, 3rd day 200,000 u/hr) (SK regimen F).

low minimum values of 0.2 to 0.3%. We might conclude from these findings that plasminogen concentrations around these values correspond to a basal plasminogen production of the organism which cannot be further lowered by a surplus of plasminogen-plasmin converting agents (Figure 17).

Fibrinogen values were rather stable under the escalating dosage regimen performed in this trial. There was a slight initial decrease from 325 mg% to 175mg% during the first 24 hr. Afterwards, the fibrinogen concentrations rose to pretreatment values (Figure 18).

VIII. LABORATORY DATA COLLECTED DURING THE INITIAL PHASE OF STREPTOKINASE TREATMENT IN PATIENTS WHO RECEIVED A LOADING DOSE EQUALING THE INDIVIDUAL CAC

In order to study the initial phase of streptokinase treatment under the above premise, three patients displaying a wide range of CAC scores, were selected.

Patient's ref. no.	CAC
605	12,000
619	490,000
620	1,000,000

In each case the titrated CAC was administered over a period of 20 min followed by a maintenance dose of 100,000 u/hr.

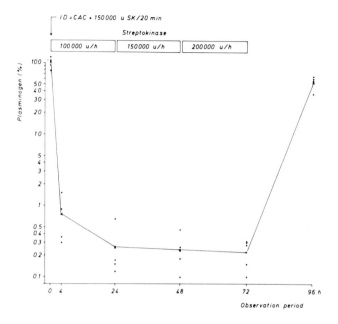

FIGURE 17.   Plasminogen concentrations in 5 patients under escalating SK inflow rates (1st day 100,000 u/hr, 2nd day 150,000 u/hr, 3rd day 200,000 u/hr) (SK regimen F).

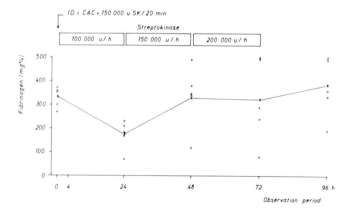

FIGURE 18.   Fibrinogen concentrations (Schulz method) in 5 patients under escalating SK inflow rates (1st day 100,000 u/hr, 2nd day 150,000 u/hr, 3rd day 200,000 u/hr) (SK regimen F).

A. Streptokinase

During the first 10 min no streptokinase activity was monitored. First streptokinase equivalents emerged after 15 to 20 min infusion time. After that, a more or less accelerated streptokinase rise was initiated (Figure 19).

B. Plasminogen

During the first 4 hr plasminogen fell steadily toward the 1% mark. Thereafter, only minor changes were recorded during the next 2 days (Figure 20).

C. Plasmin

As a rule, plasmin appeared during the 1st hr of treatment. A peak was found be-

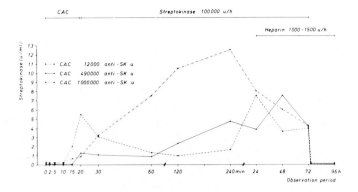

FIGURE 19.   Streptokinase concentrations in 3 patients during the initial phase of streptokinase treatment in patients who received a loading dose equaling the individual CAC.

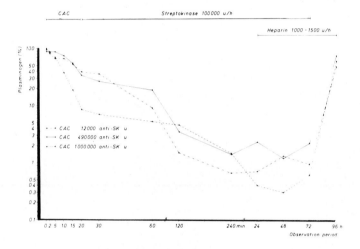

FIGURE 20.   Plasminogen concentrations in 3 patients during the initial phase of streptokinase treatment in patients who received a loading dose equaling the individual CAC.

tween the 10th and 15th min of infusion. Thereafter, plasminemia was negligible or absent over the whole period of streptokinase infusion (Figure 21).

D. Fibrinogen

Fibrinogen concentrations had their lowest level 24 hr after starting streptokinase infusion, but were severely depressed after 4 hr of treatment. The first pronounced drop was seen after 15 min, i.e., at the same point in time when a definite plasmin peak was spotted (Figure 22).

E. Partial Thromboplastin Time (PTT)

As a general feature, marked shortenings of PTT values were found at the very beginning of treatment (i.e., during the first 10 min). This speaks in favor of a transitory hypercoagulatability under streptokinase infusion, and was first described by Kappert[11] and Gross[6]. These effects had subsided after 5 min. During the following hours a definite hypocoagulatability emerged, mirroring the increasing concentration of fibrinogen degradation products. The PTT values had become normal 24 hr after start-

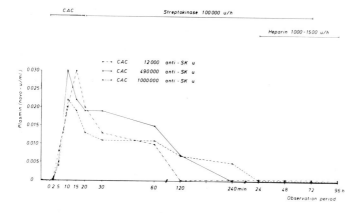

FIGURE 21.   Plasmin concentrations in 3 patients during the initial phase of streptokinase treatment in patients who received a loading dose equaling the individual CAC.

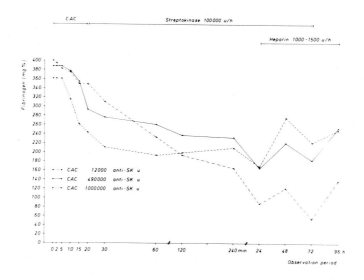

FIGURE 22.   Fibrinogen concentrations (gravimetric) in 3 patients during the initial phase of streptokinase treatment in patients who received a loading dose equaling the individual CAC.

ing treatment. Later on, PTT evaluation became impossible because of the additional heparin infusion (Figure 23).

F. Corrected Reptilase Time (cRT)

The reptilase time adjusted to a normal fibrinogen concentration reflects the coagulation-active degradation products (FDP). As can be seen in the graph of Figure 24, a marked increase in FDP was brought about between the 10th and 240th min of treatment. After 24 hr of starting therapy cRT had again normalized, thus indicating the end of anticoagulative FDP influences. At this point, an additional heparin infusion was regularly administered (Figure 24).

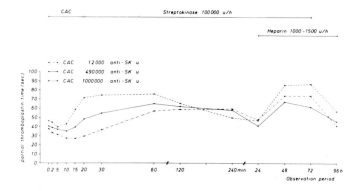

FIGURE 23.   Partial thromboplastin time (PTT) in 3 patients during the initial phase of streptokinase treatment in patients who received a loading dose equaling the individual CAC.

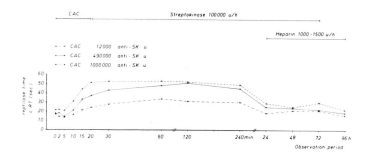

FIGURE 24.   Corrected reptilase time (cRT) in 3 patients during the initial phase of streptokinase treatment in patients who received a loading dose equaling the individual CAC.

IX. LABORATORY DATA COLLECTED DURING THE INITIAL PHASE OF STREPTOKINASE TREATMENT IN PATIENTS WHO RECEIVED A LOADING DOSE OF 250,000 U STREPTOKINASE INDEPENDENT OF THE INDIVIDUAL CAC

In order to study the initial phase of streptokinase treatment under the above premise, another three patients were selected, again displaying a wide range of CAC scores:

Patient's ref. no.	CAC
433	25,000
621	532,000
644	1,000,000

In each case, a uniform loading dose of 250,000 u/SK was infused over 20 min. Subsequently, a maintenance dose of 100,000 u SK/hr was given.

A. Streptokinase

Streptokinase concentration measured in three individuals was quite varied. A rapid streptokinase rise to 15 u/mℓ occurred in the patient with the lowest CAC value (25,000 anti-SK u) during the first 30 min of treatment. By contrast, streptokinase was unmea-

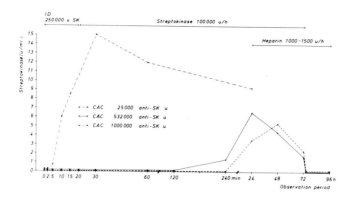

FIGURE 25.   Streptokinase concentrations in 3 patients displaying CAC
values of 25,000, 532,000 and 1,000,000 anti-SK u, respectively, who received a standard loading dose of 250,000 u SK.

surably low during the first 2 hr in the patient displaying a medium CAC value (532,000
anti-SK u). The third patient, showing a maximum CAC of 1,000,000 anti-SK u, developed no measurable streptokinase quantities at all during 4 hr of treatment, and
was still low 20 hr later (Figure 25).

B. Plasminogen

In accordance with the results of streptokinase measurements depicted above, significant plasminogen discrepancies were recorded when patients of different CAC values
were treated with the same streptokinase loading dose. In one patient, showing the
lowest CAC (25,000 anti-SK u), plasminogen fell rapidly to 0.5% during the first 10
min of treatment. In the patient displaying a medium CAC (532,000 anti-SK u), plasminogen stayed at subnormal values for about 1 hr before definitely decreasing. The
longest time lag between start of streptokinase infusion and definite plasminogen fall
was seen in the patient displaying CAC of 1,000,000 anti-SK u. Here, 4 hr passed until
a 20% decrease was monitored, and 24 hr until plasminogen fell below 3% (Figure
26).

C. Plasmin

Plasmin concentration curves in three patients receiving a schematic loading dose of
250,000 u SK in spite of varying CACs, are shown in Figure 27. Three distinct peaks
of plasmin distributed on the time axis are visible. The first peak, belonging to the
patient with the lowest CAC value, appears 5 min after starting infusion. The second
evaluation, originating from the patient with the medium range CAC, extends straight
from the 10th to the 240th min. Lastly, a 3rd peak is seen between the 2nd and 4th hr
of treatment pertaining to the patient characterized by the highest CAC value of
1,000,000 anti-SK u. Obviously, plasmin production (as well as streptokinase rise or
plasminogen fall) depends upon the ratio of CAC and loading dose. The ratio being
above 1 (i.e., loading dose larger than CAC), fibrinolytic reactions start rapidly; the
ratio being below 1 (i.e., loading dose smaller than CAC), there was a marked delay
of lytic phenomena according to the disproportion of loading dose and CAC.

D. Fibrinogen

In the low-CAC patient fibrinogen fell steeply from 420 mg% to 220 mg% during
the first 15 min of treatment (Figure 28). In contrast to this, a much slower fibrinogen
fall was found in the medium and high CAC patients. These observations of fibrinogen
concentrations reacting in accordance with CAC values point to a rule asserted earlier

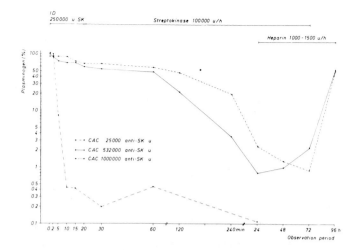

FIGURE 26. Plasminogen concentrations in 3 patients displaying CAC values of 25,000, 532,000 and 1,000,000 anti-SK u, respectively, who received a standard loading dose of 250,000 u SK.

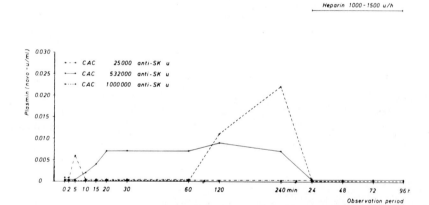

FIGURE 27. Plasmin concentrations in 3 patients displaying CAC values of 25,000, 532,000 and 1,000,000 anti-SK u, respectively, who received a standard loading dose of 250,000 u SK.

by Amery et al.[1] and Hirsh et al.[9]: relatively high loading doses (i.e., loading dose/ CAC well above 1) will produce a quicker and larger fibrinogen decrease than relatively low initial doses (i.e., loading dose/CAC well below 1).

X. LABORATORY DATA COLLECTED UPON TERMINATING STREPTOKINASE TREATMENT

Streptokinase was found to be a short-lived drug in the organism, its half-life averaging 18 min. For clinical use it is worth knowing that 1 hr after terminating infusion, only traces of streptokinase are still present in the circulation. These data tally with earlier findings of Fletcher et al.[4] and Rasche et al.[17] (Figure 29).

Plasminogen was found to be a parameter of great vivacity. Having been down to values around 0.5% under streptokinase infusion, it soars to concentrations of 1%,

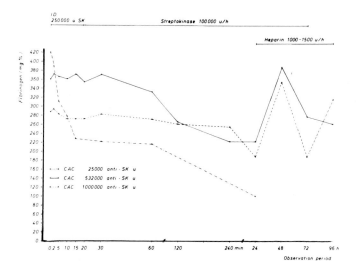

FIGURE 28.   Fibrinogen concentrations (gravimetric) in 3 patients displaying CAC values of 25,000, 532,000 and 1,000,000 anti-SK u, respectively, who received a standard loading dose of 250,000 u SK.

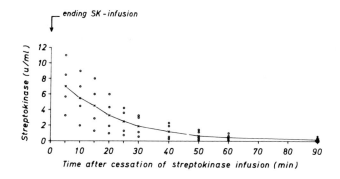

FIGURE 29.   Decrease in streptokinase concentrations after terminating 4 100,000 u/hr streptokinase treatment series.

3%, 10% and 50%, 1 hr, 2 hr, 4 hr, and 24 hr after termination of treatment (Figure 30). The plasminogen's quick rate of restoration makes checking this parameter a reliable method for monitoring streptokinase infusion. For example, a plasminogen concentration of 3% under the condition of a 100,000 u SK/hr regimen indicates an erroneous standstill of the infusion for about 2 hr.

During conventional 100,000 u SK/hr therapy *plasmin* activity rose twice between the 5th and 240th min after starting treatment (see Section III), and between the 30th min and 4th hr after termination of streptokinase treatment (Figure 31). The maximum plasmin peak was brought about 2 hr after interrupting streptokinase influx. The mechanism of plasmin regeneration after ending treatment is still tentative. However, a plasmin-forming encounter between diminishing streptokinase and rising plasminogen quantities may be involved.

XI. RELATION OF STREPTOKINASE PLASMA CONCENTRATIONS AND CAC VALUES

One streptokinase dosage scheme favored by a number of German and Swiss groups

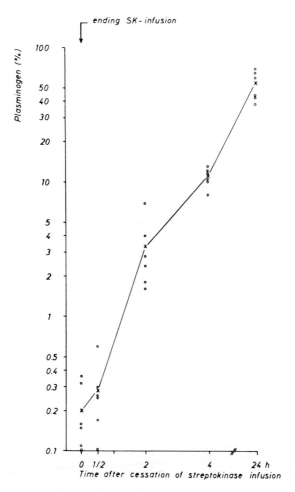

FIGURE 30. Rate of plasminogen increase after terminating
6 100,000 u/hr streptokinase treatment series.

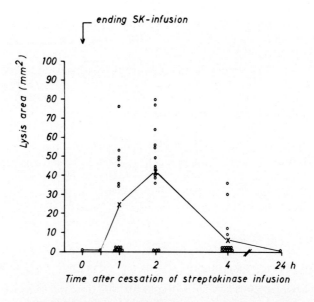

FIGURE 31. Plasmin activity upon terminating 14 100,000
u/hr streptokinase infusion series.

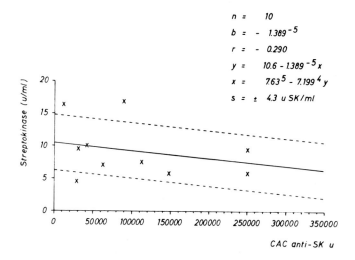

FIGURE 32.   Correlation of streptokinase plasma concentrations during streptokinase therapy and individual CACs calculated prior to streptokinase treatment; n = number of patients, b = slope of the regression line, r = correlation coefficient, x,y = formula of the regression line, s = standard deviation.

consists of an hourly streptokinase inflow rate of ⅔ of the patient's CAC. This kind of streptokinase therapy was called ''Maβlyse'' (tailored regimen) by Schmutzler[20,21].

The underlying idea was that patients displaying relatively high CACs need correspondingly high maintenance doses, and that patients showing a comparably smaller CAC required smaller maintenance doses. However, from a theoretical point of view, scarcely any arguments were brought forward sustaining this hypothesis: after administering a loading dose equaling the circulating anti-SK content (CAC) present in the patient's circulation, all anti-SK moieties are thought to be neutralized. Hence, lytic therapy will possibly start in an organism free of anti-SK, the resulting streptokinase concentration being dependent exclusively on the streptokinase inflow and its half-life in the patient.

In order to tackle this problem more thoroughly, correlation studies were carried out comparing the individual CAC values with streptokinase plasma concentrations over 3 days of treatment.

The distribution of CAC values in ten patients investigated so far were as follows:

Patient's ref. no.	CAC
584	64,000
585	147,000
591	31,000
596	242,000
598	252,000
604	112,000
605	13,000
607	48,000
609	30,000
612	89,000

The therapeutic regimen consisted of a 20 min loading dose infusion administering the calculated CAC and a 3 day maintenance dose infusion of 100,000 u SK/hr. Average

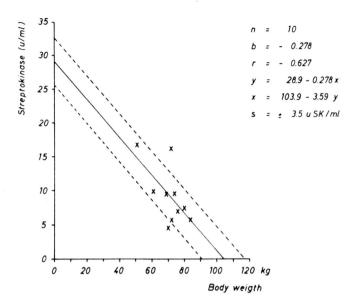

FIGURE 33. Correlation of streptokinase plasma concentration during streptokinase infusion and individual body weights; n = number of patients, b = slope of the regression line, r = correlation coefficient, x,y = formula of the regression line, s = standard deviation.

streptokinase concentrations were calculated from values determined in the plasma of each patient after 1, 2 and 3 days of treatment. Each of these average streptokinase concentrations was plotted against the individual CAC value of the respective patient.

As is shown in Figure 32, the correlation coefficient between CAC and average streptokinase concentration equaled r = −0.29, and the standard deviation was s = ± 4.3 u/mℓ. This indicates a lack of any correlation between pretreatment CACs and subsequent streptokinase plasma concentrations. According to these experimental data and the aforementioned theoretical considerations, we recommend abstaining from calculating the streptokinase maintenance doses by any given formula on the basis of pretreatment CAC values.

XII. STREPTOKINASE DOSAGE REGIMEN AND BODY WEIGHT

Ten patients were treated according to streptokinase regimen A (ID = CAC, MD = 100,000 u SK/hr). Streptokinase plasma concentrations were determined in each patient after 1, 2 and 3 days of treatment. The mean streptokinase concentrations for these 3 days were calculated and plotted vs. the individual kg body weight on a normally divided chart (Figure 33). Subsequently, the slope of the regression line, the correlation coefficient, and the standard deviation were computed.

According to the resultant data (Figure 33), no clear-cut relationship exists between the patient's body weight and the respective streptokinase concentration in his plasma. Thus, a dosage calculation based upon the patient's body weight can hardly be recommended. However, the range of body weights we dealt with in this study was relatively narrow, not going below 50 kg or exceeding 90 kg, respectively. In cases of extremely lightweight patients (e.g., children), or of abnormally heavy body weight, one must consider a reduction or an increase in the amount of streptokinase infused per hour. Accordingly, Sutor[18] recommended a loading dose in children of 4000 u SK/kg/30 min and a maintenance dose of 1000 u SK/kg/hr.

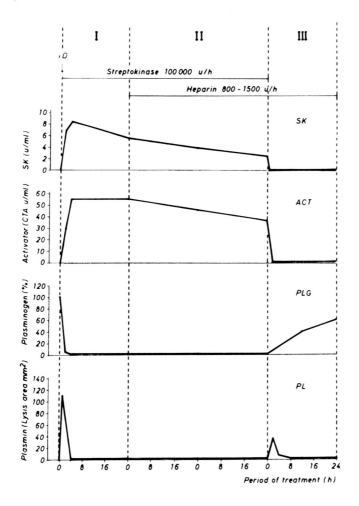

FIGURE 34.   Schematic representation of streptokinase, activator, plasminogen and plasmin concentrations during the course of a conventional streptokinase infusion regimen.

XIII. GENERAL ASSESSMENT OF SKAPPFF PATTERNS DURING STREPTOKINASE TREATMENT

In the course of, and after a conventional streptokinase application (loading dose infusion 20 min, maintenance dose infusion 100,000 u SK/hr), three different fibrinolytic reaction patterns could be distinguished (Figure 34).

During the first 24 hr period, *Phase I,* streptokinase entered the circulation, leading to concentrations of around 5 to 10 u/ml immediately after starting treatment. Concomitantly, activator climbed to a concentration of 40 to 90 CTA-u/ml. Plasminogen dropped, in a reverse manner, to 0.5% during the first 4 to 6 hr of treatment. During the first few hours a peak of plasmin was regularly traceable. Fibrinogen, by action of plasmin, broke down into fibrinogen degradation products (FDP), thus decreasing to a considerable degree.

Phase II lasted from the second day of treatment up to the point when streptokinase infusion was terminated. It was characterized by a homeostasis of low plasminogen and zero plasmin concentrations. Because of the absence of plasmin and the ensuing end of fibrinogen breakdown, there was a definite rise in fibrinogen (Figure 35). Cir-

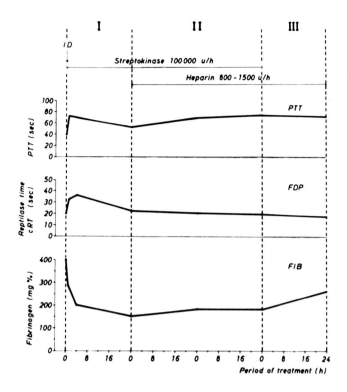

FIGURE 35. Schematic representation of the partial thromboplastin time (PTT) and the corrected reptilase time (cRT) values, as well as fibrinogen concentrations during the course of a conventional streptokinase infusion regimen.

culating FDP originating from fibrinogen degradation in Phase I of treatment had disappeared gradually, resulting in approximately normal reptilase times (cRT) (Figure 35).

Phase III covered the period of time following cessation of streptokinase infusion. Streptokinase was cleared rather quickly from the bloodstream. The half-life was found to be about 20 min. One hour after terminating streptokinase infusion, the plasma streptokinase concentration was already averaging below 0.5 u/mℓ. Since activator is composed of stoichiometric complexes of streptokinase and plasminogen (see Chapter 2), a parallel decrease in activator concentration took place.

Plasminogen recovered quickly upon terminating the streptokinase infusion, regaining values between 15 and 20% during the next 4 hr. Within 2 to 4 hr after terminating treatment, measurable quantities of plasmin were regularly found (Figure 34). A quantitative evaluation revealed that this plasmin peak was significantly less pronounced than at the beginning of treatment, and that it was not accompanied by a decrease in fibrinogen. Plasminemia, upon terminating streptokinase treatment, may be explained by transient plasminogen activation at a time when rising plasminogen was reacting with falling, but still active, streptokinase quantities.

Fibrinogen went up rather slowly (e.g., from 200 mg% at the end of infusion to 300 mg% 1 day after cessation of streptokinase inflow) (Figure 35).

Changing conventional streptokinase treatment regimen by lowering the streptokinase infusion rate to 30,000 u/hr resulted in an alteration of plasminogen-plasmin-fibrinogen behavior. Streptokinase plasma concentrations around 1 u/mℓ, as measured during this low dose regimen, were no longer able to keep plasminogen concen-

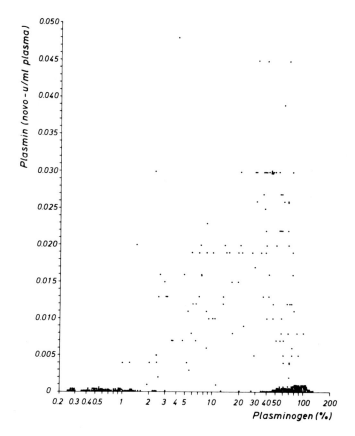

FIGURE 36.   Scattergram of plasminogen vs. plasmin as determined during various forms of streptokinase treatment.

trations as low as 0.5%, but allowed a mean plasminogen value of about 1.5%. Interestingly, this 1.5% plasminogen concentration led to plasmin activities of around 0.01 novo-u/ml throughout infusion, and to a fibrinogen level moderately lower than observed under a conventional infusion regimen. Obviously, high streptokinase concentrations were accompanied by low plasmin levels, and low streptokinase concentrations by high plasmin levels. However, reducing the amount of streptokinase infused per hour to as low a value as 5000 u SK/hr produced only a very slight plasminogen drop of about 30% and no plasmin activity at all was seen.

In order to gain a better insight into the plasminogen-plasmin relationship, a scattergram was drawn plotting plasma values (y-axis) against plasminogen concentrations (x-axis) as they were monitored during streptokinase infusion treatment. As can be seen in the chart of Figure 36, "high" (i.e., normal) and "low" (i.e., below 1%) plasminogen concentrations were found in plasma samples virtually free of plasmin. On the contrary, medium range plasminogen concentrations (i.e., between 2 to 50%) were regularly accompanied by plasmin activities of up to 0.04 novo-u/ml. Conceivably, this plasminogen/plasmin interdependence, first described by Johnson and McCarthy[10] enables the therapist, by means of adjusting the proper inflow rate, to induce a lytic treatment of either the plasmin-rich or the plasmin-poor type.

Streptokinase regimens using inflow rates above 100,000 u SK/hr were unable to induce a further decrease in plasminogen concentration below the 0.5% borderline. Obviously, the 0.5% plasminogen value must be looked on as a baseline figure maintained by the organisms' plasminogen synthesis in the presence of a concomitant plas-

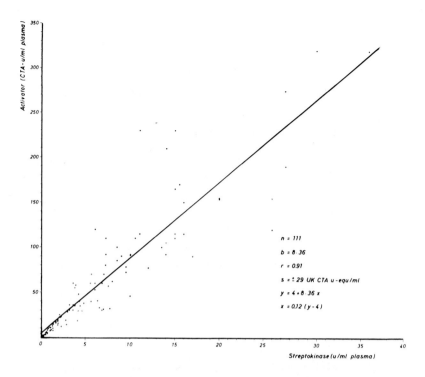

FIGURE 37. Scattergram of plasma streptokinase concentrations vs. plasma activator concentrations; both parameters were determined simultaneously during streptokinase treatment. There was a close relationship between these two parameters, the correlation coefficient equaling r = 0.91, and the slope of regression line being calculated at b = 0.8.

minogen withdrawal via plasminogen-plasmin conversion and subsequent antiplasmin neutralization.

Plasma activator activities were fully dependent on the streptokinase concentration in the plasma or on the hourly streptokinase inflow rate, respectively. Each increase in streptokinase inflow rate was mirrored by a corresponding increase in both strepto-kinase and activator concentrations, and, by the same token, a decreased streptokinase inflow rate produced a decrease in both streptokinase and activator concentrations.

To further clarify this point, streptokinase and activator concentrations determined simultaneously during streptokinase infusion were plotted one against the other, and both regression line and correlation coefficient calculated. Figure 37 shows a very close relationship between these two parameters (r = 0.91), the streptokinase/activator ratio being approximately 1:9 (SK in units/ml, activator in CTA-u/ml). Obviously, various activator concentrations (high, medium, low) can easily be arrived at by adjusting an adequate streptokinase inflow.

REFERENCES

1. **Amery, A., Donati, M. B. Vermylen, J., and Verstraete, M.,** Comparison between the changes in the plasma fibrinogen and plasminogen levels induced by a moderate or high initial dose of streptokinase, *Thrombos. Diathes. haemorrh. (Stuttg.),* 23, 504, 1970.

2. **Dotter, C. T., Rösch, J., and Seaman, A. J.,** Selective clot lysis with low dose streptokinase, *Radiology,* 111, 31, 1974.

3. **Duckert, F.,** Diskussionsbeitrag auf dem Workshop on Streptokinase der Ab Kabi, Stockholm, 1974.

4. **Fletcher, A. P., Alkjaersig, N., and Sherry, N.,** The clearance of heterologous protein from the circulation of normal and immunized man, *J. Clin. Invest.,* 37, 1306, 1958.

5. **Gallus, A. S., Hirsh, J., Cade, J. F., Turpie, A. G. G., Walker, I. R., and Gent, M.,** Thrombolysis with a combination of small doses of streptokinase and full doses of heparin, *Semin. Thromb. Hemost.,* 2, 14, 1975.

6. **Gross, R.,** Blutgerinnung und Fibrinolyse. Bericht über das II. Streptase-Kolloquium Bad Nauheim, *Behringwerk-Mitt. Heft,* 44, 1, 1964.

7. **Heikinheimo, R.,** Fibrinolysis by "Minidosage", *Curr. Ther. Res.,* 10, 382, 1968.

8. **Heikinheimo, R. and Ruosteenoja, R.,** Further experience with "Minidosage" in fibrinolytic therapy, *Curr. Ther. Res.,* 13, 444, 1971.

9. **Hirsh, J., O'Sullivan, E. F., and Martin, M.,** Evaluation of a standard dosage schedule with streptokinase, *Blood,* 35, 341, 1970.

10. **Johnson, A. J. and McCarthy, W. R.,** The lysis of artificially induced intravascular clots in man by intravenous infusions of streptokinase, *J. Clin. Invest.,* 38, 1627, 1959.

11. **Kappert, A.,** *Experimentelle Untersuchungen über Thrombogenese und Fibrinolyse,* Schwabe, Basel, 1962.

12. **Lassen, M.,** Heat denaturization of plasminogen in the fibrin plate method, *Acta Phys. Scand.,* 27, 371, 1952.

13. **Latallo, Z. S., Lopaciuk, S. and Meissner, J.,** A combined treatment with Defibrase® and streptokinase, 181—190. in *Defibrienierung mit Thrombinähnlichen Schlangengiftenzymen,* Martin, M. and Schoop, W., Eds., Verl. Hans Huber, Bern, 1975.

14. **Martin, M.,** Semiquantitative Plasminogenbestimmung mit Hilfe des Thrombelastographen. Eine Methode zur Kontrolle der Streptokinasebehandlung, *Thrombos. Diathes. haemorrh. (Stuttg.),* 22, 121, 1969.

15. **Martin, M.,** Indirect measurement of streptokinase concentration in the plasma of patients undergoing fibrinolytic treatment, *Thrombos. Diathes. Haemorrh.,* 32, 633, 1974.

16. **Martin, M.,** Studies on Activator Formation in Human Plasma with Streptokinase. III. Investigation of Activator Kinetics in Undiluted Plasma in Terms of Urokinase Equivalents, *Thrombos. Diathes. Haemorrh.,* 36, 566, 1976.

17. **Rasche, H., Hiemeyer, V., and Heimpel, H.,** Verteilungsstudien mit radioaktiv markierter Streptokinase, in *Therapeutische und experimentelle Fibrinolyse,* F. K. Schattauer Verlag, New York, 1969, 133.

18. **Sutor, A. H.,** Streptokinase treatment regimen in childhood, in *New Concepts in Streptokinase Dosimetry,* Martin, M., Schoop, W., and Hirsh, J., Eds., Hans Huber Publishers, Bern 1978.

19. **Turpie, A. G. G., Gallus, A. S., Hirsh, J., and Cade, J. F.,** Thrombolysis with a combination of small doses of streptokinase and full dose heparin, Vortrag gehalten auf dem IVth Int. Cong. Thromb. Haemost., Wien, 1973.

20. **Schmutzler, R.,** Thrombolytic treatment of acute peripheral arterial and venous occlusions, *Angiologica,* 5, 119, 1968.

21. **Schmutzler, R.,** Dosierung der thrombolytischen Therapie, in *Streptokinase Therapie bei chronischer arterieller Verschlußkrankheit,* Die Medizinische Verlagsgesellschaft mbH, Marburg, 1975, 717.

Chapter 8

ANTICOAGULANT ADMINISTRATION SUPPLEMENTARY TO STREPTOKINASE TREATMENT

I. HEPARIN AND COUMAROL ADDITION

Thrombotic events in the course of streptokinase infusion therapy, such as those reviewed in Chapter 15, in our opinion warrant anticoagulant measures both during and after fibrinolytic treatment.

Inhibition of coagulation at the start of a conventional streptokinase infusion series was regularly ensured by the appearance of appreciable amounts of fibrinogen degradation products. The inhibition rate of coagulation in terms of corrected reptilase time (cRT) and partial thromboplastin time lengthenings induced by these split products is shown in Figures 1 and 2. FDP-related inhibition of overall coagulation was present during the first 4 hr of treatment. Later on, due to subsequent decrease in FDP moieties, normal or subnormal cRT and PTT values became established. As a rule, heparin was added to streptokinase infusion at the point where cRT and PTT values approached normalcy, i.e., between the 16th and 24th hr of treatment. Immediately after starting heparin infusion, PTT values (but not the cRT which does not respond to heparin) again lengthened upward to an average value around 85 sec (normal 45 sec) and stayed there until termination of heparin inflow.

Oral coumarol medication was regularly started half a day prior to ending streptokinase infusion (Figure 3). Mostly, acenocoumarol (Sintrom®) was preferred because of its relatively brief half-life (acenocoumarol 24 hr, phenprocoumon 120 hr; Deutsch and Fischer[1], Seiler[4]). The rapid clearance of acenocoumarol was regarded as favorable with a view to checkup angiography procedures, where arterial punctures with the marked bleeding tendencies involved have to be performed. According to our experience, 1 or 2 days after termination of acenocoumarol medication the prothrombin time had already risen to values allowing arterial puncture procedures.

The acenocoumarol dosage regimen used in our patients was

- 28 mg (7 tablets) ½ day before termination of streptokinase infusion
- 48 mg (12 tablets) upon ending streptokinase infusion
- 16 mg (4 tablets) 24 hr after ending streptokinase infusion
- 8 mg (2 tablets) 48 hr after ending streptokinase infusion

The resultant prothrombin values are recorded on the graph of Figure 3.

II. DEFIBRINOGENATION PROCEDURE AS ADJUNCT TO STREPTOKINASE TREATMENT

Two effects had to be envisaged if streptokinase infusion and defibrinogenating procedures were to be combined. Firstly, fibrinogen decrease might act as a prophylactic measure for avoiding thromboembolic incidents during streptokinase infusion. Secondly, a defibrinogenation prior to streptokinase infusion possibly prevents the occurrence of large amounts of FDP normally appearing at the beginning streptokinase treatment. This might be favorable in order to counteract bleeding tendencies during that period of time.[2] However, it must be pointed out that bleeding accidents during the first 24 hr of streptokinase treatment were rarely seen.[3] Another, possibly better, rationale for introducing defibrinogenation into streptokinase treatment is the idea of

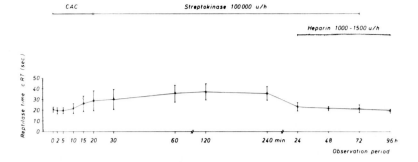

FIGURE 1.   Corrected reptilase time (cRT) is measured during a conventional streptokinase regimen according to SK regimen A. Prolonged cRT reflected the amount of
circulating FDP independent of a concomitantly decreased fibrinogen level. As could
be demonstrated, a considerable FDP amount was present in the plasma only during
the first 24 hr of treatment.

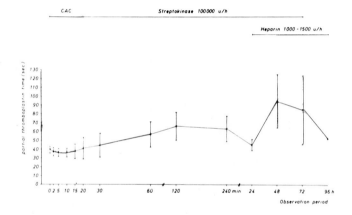

FIGURE 2.   Partial thromboplastin time (PTT) under a combined treatment with streptokinase and heparin, according to SK regimen A. After
24 hr of infusion, the PTT, having been prolonged during the first hours
of treatment, started to approach normalcy. Additional heparin infusion
was started at that point, and the PTT subsequently rose to values of
between 50 and 60 sec.

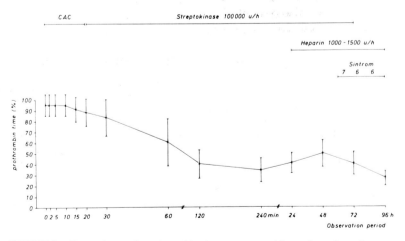

FIGURE 3.   Dependence of prothrombin times on streptokinase, heparin and acenocoumarin medication. A 30% prothrombin value was achieved on the 4th day of anticoagulant medication, consisting of a total of 76 mg acenocoumarol.

substituting heparin, a slightly fibrinolysis-inhibiting agent by an anticoagulating principle not interfering with thrombus dissolution. According to Telesforo et al.[5] heparin combines with plasma antithrombin III and thus forms a plasmin-inhibiting complex. However, this concept is highly tentative up to the present time. Clinical observations speak in favor of streptokinase-heparin treatment being an extraordinarily potent principle for in vivo clot dissolution.

In the following, some laboratory data from patients treated with a defibrinogenating drug prior to and during streptokinase infusion will be presented. The pretreatment CAC values of these five patients were:

Patient's ref. no.	CAC
D-SK 7	29,000
D-SK 8	303,000
D-SK 9	122,000
D-SK 10	59,000
D-SK 11	74,000

For use in defibrinogenation, Defibrase® (Pentapharm AG, Basel, Switzerland) was applied. The dosage regimen for combined streptokinase-Defibrase® treatment was as follows. First day: initial dose 50 $\mu\ell$/kg by 1 hr infusion (immediately before this, a single heparin injection of 20,000 u/hr was administered). Second day: start of streptokinase infusion, according to dosage regimen B. Third and fourth days: simultaneous infusion of streptokinase (100,000 u SK/hr) and Defibrase® (50 to 150 /$\mu\ell$/kg/ hr) for 24 hr each. To keep the fibrinogen level low, Defibrase® maintenance doses had to be steadily increased. Fifth day: after discontinuing streptokinase administration, treatment was perpetuated by daily Defibrase® infusions of 1 hr duration at the rate of 100 or 150 /$\mu\ell$/kg. Acenocoumarol medication started ½ day before discontinuing streptokinase inflow.

Plasminogen and fibrinogen concentration, as well as the action of fibrinogen degradation products on blood coagulation, were measured in the course of the above streptokinase-Defibrase® treatment.

Following Defibrase® pretreatment, *plasminogen* concentrations decreased by 30%. On the next day, streptokinase treatment was started with an initial plasminogen value of 70%. Under streptokinase infusion, plasminogen dropped further to values below 1% (Figure 4). The extent of this plasminogen decrease corresponded more or less to observations during streptokinase-heparin administration. By contrast, plasminogen recovery rates after cessation of streptokinase inflow turned out to be much slower under defibrinogenation than under the influence of further heparin medication. While, normally, plasminogen had already risen to values of around 50% after a 24 hr streptokinase-free interval, plasminogen still averaged 30% applying the Defibrase® modification.

Fibrinogen dropped from 387 mg% to 128 mg% in the course of Defibrase® pretreatment. Streptokinase infusion started, therefore, with a fibrinogen concentration which had been much decreased initially. Further, under combined streptokinase-Defibrase® treatment, no increase of fibrinogen was seen as it usually occurs in the course of the conventional streptokinase-heparin regimen (Figure 4).

A peak of *FDP activities* (lengthening of cRT and PTT) was monitored 4 hr after start of Defibrase® treatment. After 24 hr the subsequent streptokinase loading dose (encountering an already reduced fibrinogen level) was not followed by measurable FDP activities as was seen during streptokinase treatment without preceding defibrinogenation. Figure 5 gives the corrected reptilase times (cRT) in the course of strepto-

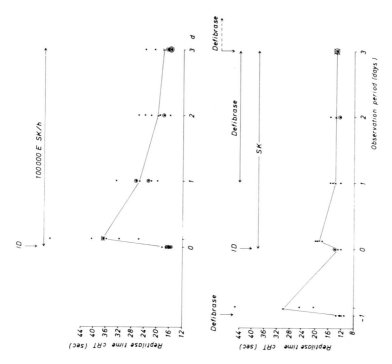

FIGURE 5.   Reptilase times corrected for fibrinogen (cRT) in the course of traditional streptokinase-heparin treatment (upper graph), and of streptokinase-Defibrase® treatment (lower graph). The cRT was thought to reflect the coagulation-active fibrinogen degradation products (FDP). It is quite obvious that in the streptokinase heparin group the main FDP peak occurred 4 hr *after* infusion of the streptokinase loading dose, whereas in the streptokinase-Defibrase® group the highest FDP concentrations were seen 24 hr *before*giving the streptokinase loading dose.

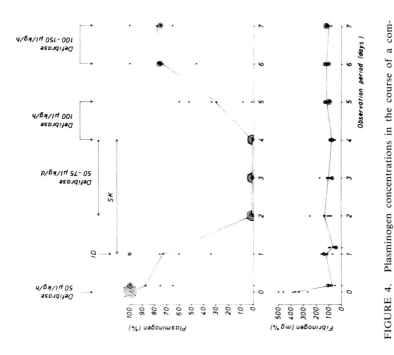

FIGURE 4.   Plasminogen concentrations in the course of a combined streptokinase-Defibrase® treatment. Fibrinogen values, concomitantly measured, are diagramed on the bottom graph.

kinase-heparin and streptokinase-Defibrase® treatment regimens, respectively. It is obvious that for the very first hours of streptokinase infusion, combined streptokinase-Defibrase® treatment was associated with a considerably smaller coagulative defect than the streptokinase-heparin regimen.

REFERENCES

1. Deutsch, E. and Fischer, M., Die Wirkung intravenös applizierter Streptokinase auf Fibrinolyse und Blutgerinnung, *Trhombos. Diathes. haemorrh. (Stuttg.),* 6, 482, 1960.
2. Latallo, Z. S. and Lopaciuk, S., New approach to thrombolytic therapy; the use of Defibrase in connection with streptokinase, *Thrombos. Diathes. haemorrh. (Stuttg.),* 56, (Suppl.) 252, 1973.
3. Martin, M., Treatment of bleeding accidents during fibrinolytic therapy, in *Reviews of Hematology,* Vol. 1, Ambrus, J. L., Ed., PJD Publ. Ltd., Westbury, N.Y., 1980.
4. Seiler, K., Entgleisung der oralen Antikoagulationbehandlung, *Schweiz. Med. Wochenschr.,* 102, 1415, 1972.
5. Telesforo, P., Semeraro, N., Verstraete, M., and Collen, D., The inhibition of plasmin by antithrombin III-heparin complex in vitro in human plasma and during streptokinase therapy in man, *Thrombos. Res.,* 7, 669, 1975.

Chapter 9

SYSTEMIC STREPTOKINASE TREATMENT OF ARTERIAL OCCLUSIONS — CLINICAL RESULTS*

This chapter reports on 475 arterial occlusions treated with streptokinase over a period of 3 days. The occlusions can be divided into 257 isolated femoral, 177 iliac, and 41 aortic obstructions. A continuous streptokinase regimen was conducted in the majority of cases. The maintenance dose applied was 100,000 u SK/hr.

I. FEMORAL OCCLUSIONS

According to the classification scheme applied in this study, a femoral occlusion involves the obstruction of the femoral artery, the popliteal artery, or both arteries. Of the 257 femoral occlusions, 217 (84%) were investigated angiographically prior to, and 121 femoral occlusions (47%) after streptokinase treatment.

The successful removal of femoral obstructions was proven angiographically in 13 out of 20 cases (65%). Clinical diagnostic methods, as described in chapter 6, were applied to the rest of the contingent.

The group of femoral occlusions had to be subdivided because, aside from 225 chronic occlusions, there were 32 occlusions of nonchronic origin, such as reocclusions after transluminal catheter treatment, or vascular surgery and thrombotic accidents following catheter angiography.

The successful removal of chronic femoral blockings was possible in 8.9% (20/225) (Figure 1). Looking at the history of femoral occlusions, it became evident that there was a close relationship between the clearance rate of femoral arteries and the age of the femoral occlusions. For example, 97% (198/205) of the nonresponders (no lytic success) had a claudication history of more than 6 weeks, whereas in the responder group (streptokinase treatment led to opening of the femoral artery) only 25% (5/20) displayed such a long occlusion time.

In focusing more thoroughly on the occlusion time vs. success rate, the following data were compiled. In patients undergoing lysis treatment during the very first 2 weeks after femoral occlusion, a clearance was established in 75% (12/16). Femoral occlusions of 2 to 6 weeks standing showed a 57% (4/7) removal rate, i.e., the success rate was slightly reduced compared with the 2-week history group. A 38% clearance rate (3/8) of 6-week to 3-month-old femoral occlusions seemed relatively low compared with the femoral occlusions of shorter standing. Femoral occlusions older than 6 months were virtually nonlysable. Angiograms prior to and after successfully conducted streptokinase treatment in chronic femoral occlusions are compiled in Figures A-1 to A-4 in the Appendix section of this book.

II. LYTIC TREATMENT OF FEMORAL OCCLUSIONS AFTER VASCULAR SURGERY AND TRANSLUMINAL CATHETER PROCEDURES

In the course of lytic treatment 33% (5/15) of femoral arteries** which reoccluded 2 to 40 months after vascular surgery reopened again (Table 1). As in the chronic

---

* Some paragraphs in this chapter have been prepublished by M. Martin in *Progr. Cardiovasc. Dis.*, 21, 5, 1979. We thank Grune & Stratton for the permission to reprint these items.

** As mentioned earlier, the popliteal artery was classified as part of the distal femoral artery.

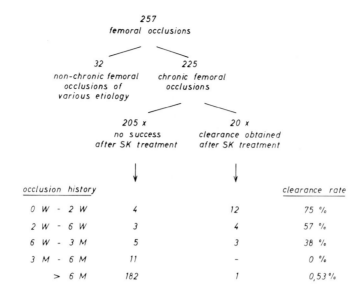

257
femoral occlusions

32
non-chronic femoral
occlusions of
various etiology

225
chronic femoral
occlusions

205 x
no success
after SK treatment

20 x
clearance obtained
after SK treatment

occlusion history			clearance rate
0 W - 2 W	4	12	75 %
2 W - 6 W	3	4	57 %
6 W - 3 M	5	3	38 %
3 M - 6 M	11	-	0 %
> 6 M	182	1	0,53 %

FIGURE 1.   Diagram of lytic results in streptokinase treatment of femoral occlusions in relation to the occlusion history.

Table 1
COMPILATION OF DATA ON PATIENTS TREATED BY STREPTOKINASE INFUSION AFTER FEMORAL REOCCLUSION FOLLOWING VASCULAR SURGERY

Patient ref. no.	Side	Type of vascular surgery prior to occlusion	Period between arterial surgery and reocclusion	Period between reocclusion and lytic treatment	Success of lytic treatment
82	Right	Thromboendarterectomy	24 months	16 hours	+
129	Right	Thromboendarterectomy	4 months	4 months	Ø
182	Left	Thromboendarterectomy	?	5 weeks	Ø
215	Left	Thromboendarterectomy	6months	3 days	+
227	Right	Venous bypass	9 months	3 weeks	Ø
279	Left	Thromboendarterectomy	?	?	Ø
392	Right	Venous bypass	6 months	6 weeks	Ø
402	Right	Thromboendarterectomy	7 months	1 day	Ø
405	Right	Thromboendarterectomy	11 months	17 days	+
423	Left	Venous bypass	2 months	20 days	Ø
507	Left	Thromboendarterectomy	40 months	1 year	Ø
514	Left	Thromboendarterectomy	33 months	4 weeks	+
515	Left	Venous bypass	8 months	3 weeks	Ø
516	Right	Thromboendarterectomy	?	1 year	Ø
528	Right	Thromboendarterectomy	26 months	10 days	+

group, lytic success was closely related to the occlusion age. Streptokinase treatment carried out on 10 patients 6 days to 4 weeks after transluminal catheter treatment according to Dotter[1] (percutaneous transluminal angioplasty = PTA), during which an immediate reocclusion was recorded, led to clearance in 30% (3/10) (Table 2). Thrombotic or embolic occlusions of arteries developing in the course of angiographic procedures were treated 5 to 10 days after the incident. A 43% (3/7) dissolution of these obstructions was possible (Table 3).

Table 2

COMPILATION OF DATA ON PATIENTS TREATED BY STREPTOKINASE
INFUSION AFTER FEMORAL REOCCLUSION FOLLOWING CATHETER
TREATMENT ACCORDING TO DOTTER[1]

Patient ref. no.	Side	Result of catheter treatment	Standing of occlusion prior to catheter treatment	Success of lytic treatment
188	Right	Occlusion mass was penetrated but patency not achieved	14 days	Ø
228	Left	Clearance was achieved but reocclusion set in during the next hours	4 weeks	Ø
312	Left	Occlusion mass was penetrated but patency not achieved	4 weeks	Ø
411	Left	Occlusion mass was penetrated but patency not achieved	15 days	+
429	Right	Clearance was achieved but reocclusion set in during the next hours	6 days	Ø
436	Left	Occlusion mass was penetrated but patency not achieved	12 days	+
452	Right	Occlusion mass was penetrated but patency not achieved	13 days	Ø
464	Right	Clearance was achieved but reocclusion set in during the next hours	4 weeks	Ø
503	Left	Occlusion mass was penetrated but patency not achieved	20 days	Ø
578	Left	Occlusion mass was penetrated but patency not achieved	4 weeks	+

Table 3

COMPILATION OF DATA ON PATIENTS WHO
DEVELOPED ACUTE FEMORAL OCCLUSION
AFTER ANGIOGRAPHIC PROCEDURES AND
WHO WERE SUBSEQUENTLY TREATED BY
STREPTOKINASE INFUSION

Patient ref. no.	Side	Period between occlusion and lytic treatment	Success of lytic treatment
20	Left	5 days	+
221	Left	7 days	Ø
269	Right	15 days	Ø
393	Right	13 days	Ø
413	Left	11 days	Ø
498	Right	10 days	+
592	Right	9 days	+

III. ILIAC OCCLUSIONS

Iliac occlusions in 177 patients underwent a 3 day streptokinase treatment. The largest part, namely 169 cases (96%), reflected the natural course of the chronic arterial occlusion disease. In another 4 cases the occlusion incident occurred 1 to 38 months after vascular surgery, and in another 4 cases iliac occlusions were connected with angiographic catheter procedures. Of the 177 iliac arteries, 168 (95%) were investigated angiographically prior to, and 70 iliac arteries (40%) after streptokinase treatment.

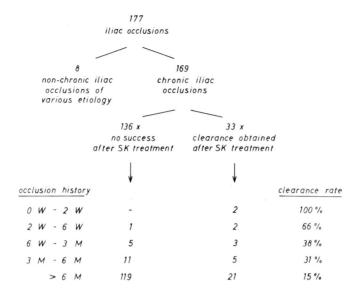

FIGURE 2.   Diagram of lytic results in streptokinase treatment of iliac
occlusions in relation to the occlusion history.

"Iliac occlusion" was defined as an occlusion of the common iliac artery, the external iliac artery, or both the common and external iliac arteries.

In the course of the 3 day streptokinase treatment, complete dissolution of the iliac thrombus masses had been achieved in 33 of the 169 chronic occlusions (20%) (Figure 2). Of these 33 cases, 17 (52%) were controlled by means of angiographic methods, the rest with the help of clinical procedures (pulse taking, auscultation, oscillogram, ultrasonic pressure measurement. See Chapter 6.)

As in the femoral group, there was a striking relationship between the average occlusion times and the respective clearance rates. Best lytic results were achieved if the history of iliac occlusion was well below 3 months duration. Here, an opening rate of 46% (6/13) was recorded (Figure 2). Later on, the clearance rate fell to less favorable values. For example, iliac occlusions of 3 to 6 months standing had a lysis rate of no more than 31%. Iliac occlusions older than 6 months displayed a 15% removal rate and therefore were not suited for lytic treatment from the clinical point of view. Angiograms prior to and after successfully conducted streptokinase treatment are compiled in the Appendix Section, Figures A-5 to A-10. Iliac occlusions of types other than chronic obstruction are compiled in Tables 4 and 5. Four iliac arteries that had reoccluded 1 to 38 months after vascular surgery underwent a subsequent streptokinase treatment 20 days to 7 weeks thereafter. The clearance rate was 75% (3/4). In another four cases, fresh iliac thrombosis occurred during or immediately after catheter arteriography. Streptokinase treatment was carried out 10 days to 8 weeks later, leading again to a clearance rate of 75% (3/4).

In another attempt both the common iliac and the external iliac occlusions were looked at separately. This was possible in the group of 168 cases where angiography was performed prior to treatment. It can be seen on the graph of Figures 3 and 4 that the lytic results in both the common and external iliac occlusions are fairly comparable to clearance rates in the overall iliac artery group. On the other hand, due to the rarity of combined common and external iliac occlusions, no definite statement regarding the clearance rate can be made (Figure 5).

Table 4
COMPILATION OF LYTIC RESULTS IN STREPTOKINASE-TREATED ILIAC ARTERIES REOCCLUDED AFTER VASCULAR SURGERY

Patient ref. no.	Location	Type of vascular surgery prior to occlusion	Period between surgery and reocclusion	Period between reocclusion and lytic treatment	Success of lytic treatment
334	Left common iliac artery	Thromboendarterectomy	5 months	4 weeks	Ø
416	Left external iliac artery	Thromboendarterectomy	1 month	20 days	+
472	Left common iliac artery	Aortic bifurcation prothesis	36 months	6 weeks	+
554	Right common iliac artery	Thromboendarterectomy	38 months	7 weeks	+

Table 5
COMPILATION OF LYTIC RESULTS IN STREPTOKINASE-TREATED ILIAC ARTERIES THROMBOSED IN THE COURSE OF ANGIOGRAPHIC PROCEDURES

Patient ref. no.	Location	Period between occlusion and lytic treatment	Success of lytic treatment
238	Right common iliac artery	27 days	+
239	Right common iliac artery	8 weeks	+
568	Left external iliac artery	10 days	Ø
597	Right external iliac artery	14 days	+

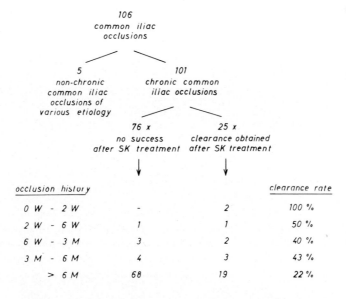

FIGURE 3.   Diagram of lytic results in streptokinase treatment of common iliac occlusions in relation to the occlusion history.

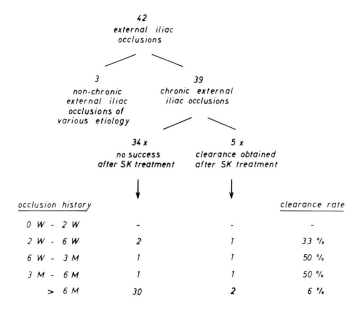

FIGURE 4.   Diagram of lytic results in streptokinase treatment of external iliac occlusions in relation to the occlusion history.

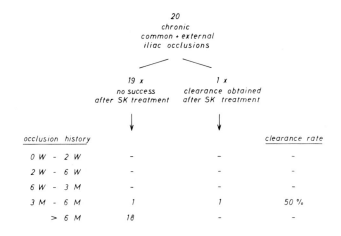

FIGURE 5.   Diagram of lytic results in streptokinase treatment of combined common and external iliac occlusions in relation to the occlusion history.

IV. AORTIC OCCLUSIONS

Aortic occlusions (41 cases) were treated by a 2 day streptokinase infusion. In this context aortic occlusions are defined as occlusions of the abdominal aorta, with or without a concomitant bilateral iliac occlusion. In each case an angiogram was carried out before treatment, and also in 15 cases after ending therapy. Checkup angiography in the group where removal of the obstruction had been possible, was performed in 70%.

Streptokinase treatment was capable of removing the aortic obstruction in 24% (10/41) (Figure 6). Since only four patients had a history of aggravated claudication pain during the last 6 months, no further investigation of the occlusion time vs. clearance

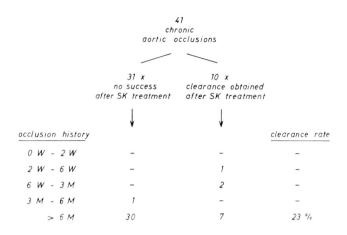

FIGURE 6.   Diagram of lytic results in streptokinase treatment of chronic aortic occlusions in relation to the occlusion history.

rate relationship was conducted. It must be pointed out, however, that longstanding obstructions beyond the 6 month borderline were removed in 23% (7/30). For angiograms taken prior to and after successfully conducted lytic treatment.

It seems worth mentioning that during streptokinase treatment of a subrenal aortic obstruction, the inferior pole artery of the right kidney became occluded. Subsequently, a marked decrease in renal function evolved, leading to creatine concentrations of up to 2.2 mg%. This incident might have been due to multiple microemboli being chipped off from the aortic thrombus, leading to microembolism in both kidneys. Therefore, in subrenal aortic occlusions we would give streptokinase treatment only in those cases where vascular surgery can not be carried out on the grounds of coronary heart disease, freak constitution, etc.

V. PERIOD OF LYTIC TREATMENT DURING WHICH CLEARANCE OF FORMERLY OCCLUDED ARTERIES WAS ACHIEVED

The exact point in time at which complete lysis of an arterial occlusion occurred was investigated in 55 successfully treated patients. Methods for evaluating patency were daily oscillography at rest and after exercise, measurement of ankle pressure, and routine clinical examination (pulse taking, auscultation). Streptokinase treatment lasted 3 days in every one of the 55 patients tested. As is seen in the graph of Figure 7, 40% of the vessels were cleared after a treatment period of 24 hr, another 40% after a period of 48 hr, and 16% after 3 days of streptokinase treatment. Furthermore, 4% of the occluded arteries opened *after* cessation of streptokinase infusion.

These figures indicate that the clearance rate of arteries under lytic treatment declined constantly over the whole period of treatment. We would recommend, therefore, not to extend lytic therapy of arterial occlusions beyond a 3 day period.

Of great interest was the finding that 4% of successfully treated arterial occlusions opened one or more days *after* termination of streptokinase infusion. The mechanism behind this finding is still unclear. However, thrombolytic reactions on the surface of a thrombus soaked with considerable amounts of streptokinase, and at the same time surrounded by blood displaying rising concentrations of plasminogen, may play a part.

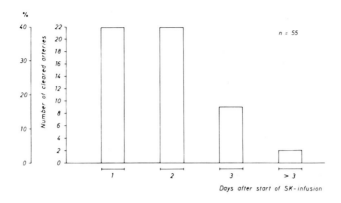

FIGURE 7.   Time of streptokinase therapy in patients with successful resolution of chronic arterial occlusions until first improvements appeared.

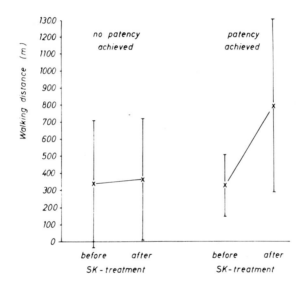

FIGURE 8.   Difference in walking capability before and after streptokinase treatment. On the left side, pre- and post-treatment walking distances measured in patients in whom vessel patency could not be achieved (no lengthening of walking distance). On the right side, pre- and post-treatment walking distances measured in patients in whom clearance of a formerly occluded artery was possible (increase in walking distance). Walking distance was determined at 120 steps/min.

VI. RELATIONSHIP OF VESSEL CLEARANCE RATE AND WALKING DISTANCE

The point was made earlier (Kaindl et al.[2]) that lengthening of walking distance was frequently seen after streptokinase treatment, even in cases where no vessel clearance was achieved. The rationale behind this finding might have been that patients who underwent the strenuous and impressive experience of fibrinolytic procedures were not inclined to admit that this treatment could be a failure. However, as these conclusions were drawn from only 7 patients, we initiated a retrospective study investigating the walking distances before and after streptokinase treatment in a group of 11 patients where vessel clearance had been achieved, and in another group of 19 patients where no such success was recorded. In each case the claudication history was less than 3 months. Occlusion sites were femoral and iliac arteries. In every case the walking test was performed at a frequency of 120 steps/min as controlled by a metronome. The results are summarized in Figure 8. As can be seen from this chart, there was no lengthening in walking distance of patients where streptokinase treatment had failed (no vessel clearance obtained). On the other hand, a significant average rise in walking distance, from 325 up to 800 m (p < 0.05) was seen when vessel clearance had been recorded.

In considering these facts it seems mandatory that vessel patency is the sole target of lytic treatment. This, in turn, urges the therapist to abide by a list of clearly defined indications guaranteeing a maximum rate of vessel clearance.

REFERENCES

1. Dotter, C. T. and Judkins, M. P., Transluminal treatment of arteriosclerotic obstruction: description of a new technique and a preliminary report of its application, *Circulation,* 30, 654, 1964.
2. Kaindl, F., Pilgerstorfer, H. W., Weidinger, P., and Fischer, M., Untersuchungen zur Thrombolyse alterer arterieller Verschlusse mit Streptokinase, *Med. Welt.,* 1713, 1968.

Chapter 10

SYSTEMIC STREPTOKINASE TREATMENT OF ARTERIAL NARROWINGS — CLINICAL RESULTS*

An arterial stenosis that affects blood flow because of thrombotic deposits on the vascular wall is a particularly appropriate model for testing the effectiveness of thrombolytic treatment. Even the smallest changes in the caliber of the lumen cause hemodynamic effects which become apparent in both the ankle pressure measurement and oscillogram after exercise.

In earlier publications based on the results of 102 arterial stenoses in 96 patients (Martin et al.[4]), a definite widening of aortic stenoses was recorded in 75%, of common iliac stenoses in 59%, of external iliac stenoses in 53%, and of femoral stenoses in 20%. In most of these cases a 3 day, 100,000 u SK/hr treatment regimen was carried out. An angiogram was performed in each patient before streptokinase treatment and a control angiography was performed in 37 of 50 stenoses listed as successfully widened. It soon became evident that primarily short stenoses of a crumbly, rough, and uneven shape located in relatively wide vessels, such as aorta or iliac arteries, were best amenable to lysis.

Bearing in mind these preliminary observations, another attempt was made to investigate more extensively the ratio of stenosis morphology vs. the extent of widening during streptokinase treatment. This study covered 47 iliac stenoses without additional obstructions upstream or downstream.

Poststenotic systolic ankle pressure measurements in the posterior tibial arteries were performed prior to, during, and after treatment. All measurements were conducted by adopting the ultrasonic technique (see Chapter 6). According to the results of measurement relatively narrow stenoses displayed a rather low ankle pressure, whereas wider stenoses showed a much higher ankle pressure. Lytic results could easily be monitored by determining the ankle pressure before and after streptokinase treatment. The widening of an arterial stenosis was always signaled by an increase in the ankle pressure figures.

Upon further analysis it was confirmed that some, but not all, narrowings responded favorably to streptokinase treatment. In order to arrive at a scheme by which the therapeutic response could be predicted, data for several types of narrowings responding differently to streptokinase treatment were compiled. The principle of classification was based on morphological details derived from the angiogram. One large group, consisting of rough, irregular or granular forms, was coded Types A to C (Figure 1 and A-14, A-17 to A-20, A-22 to A-24). As could be demonstrated by ankle pressure measurements and angiograms, these forms were specifically amenable to lysis. The pretreatment and posttreatment ankle pressure values averaged 89 and 123 mmHg each (Figure 2). In contrast to this, smooth and streamlined narrowings, coded Types M to P (Figure 1 and A-26 to A-29 in the Appendix), were fully resistant to streptokinase treatment (no change or even a decrease in posttreatment ankle pressure). Small, translucent recesses of irregular shape in otherwise unaltered vessel segments, coded Type K (Figure A-21), also responded favorably. However, the case number of this latter group was too small for statistical evaluation.

The above findings indicate that surface analysis must be regarded as a necessary prerequisite for obtaining satisfactory results in widening arterial stenoses by strepto-

---

* Some paragraphs in this chapter have been prepublished by M. Martin in *Progr. Cardiovasc. Dis.*, 21, 5, 1979. We thank Grune & Stratton for the permission to reprint these items.

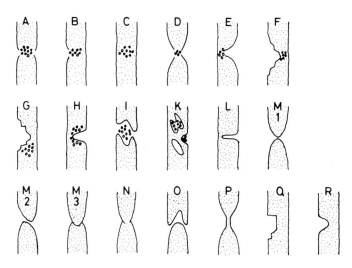

FIGURE 1.   A schematic representation of 19 different types of stenoses, coded A to R, in the common iliac artery.

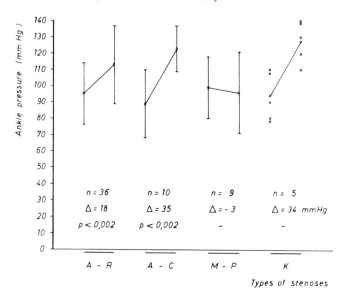

FIGURE 2.   Narrowings of the common iliac artery in 60 patients were investigated by use of the ultrasonic pressure measurement technique before and after streptokinase treatment. Stenoses types A through D and K (see Figure 1) responded favorably to lysis (rise in ankle pressure from 89 to 123 mmHg). Types M through P were unaffected by lytic therapy.

kinase treatment. X-ray analysis of arterial stenoses must be looked upon as an indispensable tool for predicting the therapeutic outcome of treatment.

As to the period of time required for widening stenoses by fibrinolytic treatment 23 narrowings were investigated (Figure 3). In 70% a widening was perceptible 1 day after initiation of treatment. A further 17% was widened after 2 days of therapy, another 9% after 3 days, and 4% after terminating treatment.

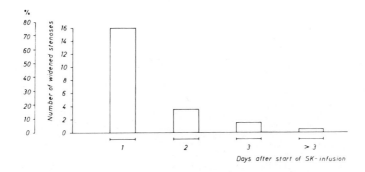

FIGURE 3.   Time of streptokinase therapy until definite improvement appeared in patients in which stenoses were widened successfully.

REFERENCE

1. **Martin, M., Schoop, W., and Zeitler, E.**, Streptokinase in chronic arterial occlusive disease, *JAMA*, 211, 1169, 1970.

Chapter 11

VARIATIONS IN STREPTOKINASE REGIMEN SCHEMES — CLINICAL RESULTS

I. INFUSION OF STREPTOKINASE INTO THROMBUS MATERIAL ("CATHETER LYSIS")

In 1974, a paper was presented by Dotter et al.[1] holding that streptokinase infusion into the arterial occlusion might be a reliable method for clearing arteries obstructed by thrombus material. In a subsequent study carried out by our group, 6 patients displaying femoral occlusions of 15 to 20 cm in length were treated according to the scheme given by the above authors. The claudication history of these patients varied between 8 weeks and 18 months.

The single steps were as follows. The common femoral artery was punctured in the groin. A Teflon® French 6 catheter was inserted into the superficial femoral artery, the tip being placed in the middle of the occlusion mass. The catheter was prepared prior to treatment so as to have five small outlets situated around the open-ended tip. After insertion, the catheter was fixed to the skin of the groin. In most instances, a distinct backflow was recorded immediately after inserting the catheter. The proximal catheter outlet was attached to the infusion pump, allowing the administration of the streptokinase loading dose (equivalent of the circulating CAC dissolved in 20 mℓ 5% glucose solution) over 20 min, and subsequently of the maintenance dose of 5000 u SK/hr (dissolved in 2 mℓ glucose solution) over 24 hr (see Figure 1). As pointed out before, all streptokinase solutions were instilled directly into the arterial occlusion masses. Yet, judging from the immediate backflow after insertion of the catheter, a free connection between the circulating blood and the catheter's tip (probably via perforated thrombus material) has to be anticipated.

Together with streptokinase administration, a heparin infusion of 1000 u heparin/hr was administered intravenously (cubital vein). This anticoagulant measure was thought necessary for preventing thrombus adhesion to the wall of the catheter being placed in the artery's cavity. After termination of the 24 hr combined I.V. heparin/I.A. streptokinase infusion, a checkup angiogram was performed and the Teflon® catheter removed. The aftertreatment consisted of I.V. heparin infusion and acenocoumarol medication.

Judging from both the checkup angiograms and the results of clinical investigations (pulse taking, ascultation, oscillography, ultrasonic pressure measurement) removal of four of the six chronic femoral occlusions was achieved (Table 1) (Figures A-30 to A-34, in the Appendix). So far, streptokinase infused directly into longstanding (several months) and fairly extended (20 to 25 cm in length) femoral occlusions might be a reasonable alternative to other therapeutic measures. However, long-term intraarterial infusions include some risks that call for scrupulous surveillance of the patients. The connection between infusion pump and the proximal end of the catheter has to fit closely. Disconnection would lead immediately to a considerable loss of blood (arterial bleeding). Further, a concomitant intravenous heparin infusion parallel to the streptokinase administration was a necessary prophylactic measure in order to avoid fresh thrombus adhesion to the catheter surface during the period of treatment (see Appendix, Figure A-31). Thrombus material adhering to the catheter surface will inevitably be stripped off during catheter withdrawal. In one of the five cases presented in this trial, a distinct thrombus layer had developed during a 6 hr standstill of the heparin infusion pump (Figure 1). After removal of the catheter, the thrombus masses re-

Table 1
COMPILATION OF DATA PERTAINING TO PATIENTS TREATED BY CATHETER LYSIS

Patient	Age (years)	Location	History of occlusion	Clearance
485	50	Right femoral a. occlusion	6 months	+
487	59	Right femoral a. occlusion	9 months	+
488	58	Right femoral a. occlusion	6 months	+
489	59	Right femoral a. occlusion	18 months	+
495	65	Left femoral a. occlusion	2 months	+
497	54	Right femoral a. occlusion	7 months	ø

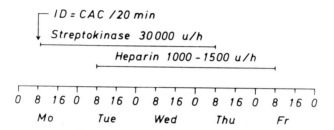

FIGURE 1.   Low dosage regimen schedule. The loading dose (ID) equaled the CAC. The maintenance dose was 30,000 u SK/hr administered over a period of 72 hr. Starting with second day of treatment, heparin overlapped with streptokinase and continued alone after cessation of streptokinase.   Heparin was withdrawn if the prothrombin time, lengthened by acenocoumarol medication (Sintrom®), reached the therapeutic level of below 25%.

mained in the vessel and were shown to cover the internal surface of the artery. Fortunately, the masses neither occluded the lumen nor embolized into deeper parts of the circulation. However, this incident clearly emphasized the need for efficient anticoagulative measures during the 24 hr management of catheter lysis.

II. INTERMITTENT DOSAGE REGIMEN

Intermittent streptokinase dosage regimen consisted of a 2 day streptokinase infusion period, followed either by a 16 hr SK/free interval and another 12 hr SK infusion; or by a 24 hr SK/free interval and another 24 hr SK infusion. The reason for conducting intermittent streptokinase treatment was twofold: to increase the number of periods rich in circulating plasmin (each 100,000 u/hr SK infusion series started and ended with a marked plasminemia), and to enlarge the number of periods characterized by normal or subnormal plasma plasminogen concentration (which was below 1% during, but rose immediately to appreciable levels after interruption of SK influx).

As plasminemia is thought to ensure a frontal, exogenous clot lysing effect,[6] multiple periods of plasminemia were estimated as possibly being a valuable adjunct to an otherwise plasmin-free conducted treatment. Further, according to Gottlob and Blümel[5],

Table 2
PERIOD OF TIME DURING WHICH OCCLUSIONS WERE REMOVED OR STENOSES WIDENED IN THE COURSE OF INTERMITTENT STREPTOKINASE TREATMENT

	Removal of occlusions	Widening of stenosis
No improvement	19	15
Improvement at unknown time	—	1
Improvement during first infusion series	4	9
Improvement immediately after first infusion series	2	2
Improvement 12 hr after ending first infusion series	1	—
Improvement immediately after second infusion series	2	—
Improvement 12 hr after ending second infusion series	1	1

Note: As is seen, 3 of 10 successfully treated occlusions, and 1 of 13 widened stenoses improved during or after the second infusion series.

SK-impregnated thrombi would rapidly lyse in media of high plasminogen concentrations. During the intermittent regimen, these obviously effective mechanisms were put into effect by interposing a streptokinase-free pause between the first and second streptokinase infusion series, thus allowing plasminogen to rise again and to combine with streptokinase on the clot surface, leading to additional lytic effects.

In Chapter 7 the respective laboratory figures (plasma streptokinase, plasminogen, plasmin, and activator concentrations) are compiled and discussed extensively.

The results of intermittent streptokinase treatment are compiled in Table 2. The percentage of vessel clearance and stenoses widening turned out to be at about the same rate as during continuous treatment. First signs of improvement were recorded during or immediately after the first 2-day continuous part of treatment in the majority of cases. However, three occlusions dissolved and one stenosis widened during or after the second series of SK infusion. This would at least point to the usefulness of this regimen. Yet, the superiority of the intermittent scheme has not yet been proven and can be established only by controlled trials comprising a much larger number of patients than was shown here.

III. SMALL DOSAGE REGIMEN FOR WIDENING ARTERIAL STENOSES

Recently, there have been several reports on successful lytic therapy of arterial or venous occlusions using streptokinase regimens with hourly doses well below 100,000 u (Turpie et al.[8]: 5000 to 20,000 u/hr; Duckert[2]: 10,000 u/hr; Latallo et al.[7]: 10,000 to 20,000 u/hr; Gallus et al.[4]: 10,000 u/hr). Yet, up to now, no account of small dosage regimens in arterial stenoses has been made available. The following paragraphs present a study aimed at answering the question of whether low dose streptokinase treatment may or may not be looked upon as a potent means for widening iliac stenoses.

A total of 10 patients displaying 13 arterial stenoses (10 common iliac artery, 1 external iliac artery, 1 aortic bifurcation) were treated. All stenoses showed a crumbly, irregular shape known to be especially suited for lysis (see Chapter 10). The length of the narrowings ranged from 0.5 to 3 cm (Table 3). The treatment consisted of a 3 day 30,000 u SK/hr scheme (Figure 2). Each treatment series started by administration of a loading dose equaling the individual CAC (circulating anti-SK content). Subsequently, a maintenance dose of 30,000 u SK/hr was infused. In all patients an angiogram was at hand prior to treatment, during treatment, and after termination of treatment. Laboratory parameters controlled were plasma streptokinase concentration, plasminogen, plasmin, fibrinogen and PTT.

A. Clinical Results

Prior to treatment, the average ankle pressure of the patient group was recorded at 80 mmHg. One day after conclusion of therapy, the ankle pressure had increased to 104 mmHg (Figure 2; Table 3). The rise in poststenotic systolic pressure was statistically significant at $p < 0.0005$ (Wilcoxon matched-pairs signed-ranks test).

First signs of widening, as recorded by means of oscillography and ultrasonic Doppler technique, were seen in 2 patients after 24 hr and in 10 patients after 48 hr of treatment. No improvement was found in 1 patient with a common iliac narrowing. Changes in the fibrinolytic parameters (SK concentration, plasminogen, plasmin, fibrinogen) during the 30,000 u SK/hr regimen are depicted in Figures 8, 9, and 10 of Chapter 7. The most characteristic features were a moderately lowered plasminogen and fibrinogen concentration and a measurable plasminemia throughout infusion.

B. Comments

The data accumulated in the course of low dosage streptokinase therapy showed a significant widening of arterial stenoses. However, the periods of lysis time up to the point where first improvements became measurable differed largely in the groups of low dosage and conventional dosage regimens. As is apparent from Table 3, after 24 hr infusion 16.7% of the stenoses became wider in the low dosage regimen group, whereas 50% became wider in the conventional group after the same period of time. This difference is indicative of the view that a low dosage regimen might be less effective than a larger one, or, in other words, that in order to achieve a defined lytic effect, relatively long periods of low dosage streptokinase infusion are necessary, compared to relatively short periods of conventional streptokinase infusions.

A further point concerns the cerebral accident rate. In another low dosage streptokinase coronary trial not yet published by our group, one fatal cerebral bleeding was recorded on the second day of treatment. Gallus et al.[4] likewise reported on a lethal intracerebral hemorrhage on the 5th day of combined 20,000 u SK/hr heparin treatment. From this one might conclude that low dosage SK treatment cannot be considered safer than the conventional kind of SK administration (100,000 u SK/hr).

It certainly would be worthwhile to compare both clinical benefits and bleeding accidents in the two groups on a randomized and double-blind basis.

Table 3
COMPILATION OF CLINICAL DATA BEFORE AND AFTER A LOW DOSAGE STREPTOKINASE TREATMENT IN 10 PATIENTS DISPLAYING 13 ILIAC OR AORTIC STENOSES

Patient ref. no.	Age (years)	Initial dose (u SK)	Location	Length of stenoses	Ankle pressure (mmHg)		Period of time after which first signs of stenosis widening were recorded
					Prior to therapy	After therapy	
527	57	150,000	Left ext. iliac	8 mm	80	140	24 hr
531	48	150,000	Right comm. iliac	5 mm	110	120	48 hr
538	53	75,000	Right comm. iliac	7 mm	80	130	24 hr
539	52	25,000	Right aortic bifurcation	7 mm	60	90	48 hr
			Left aortic bifurcation	7 mm	60	90	48 hr
543	53	75,000	Right comm. iliac	11 mm	90	110	48 hr
			Left comm. iliac	6 mm	70	80	48 hr
			Left femoral a. occlusion				
561	54	250,000	Left comm. iliac	30 mm	90	70	—
564	54	200,000	Right comm. iliac	5 mm	100	120	48 hr
566	54	450,000	Left comm. iliac	10 mm	100	140	48 hr
572	51	200,000	Right comm. iliac	5 mm	60	80	48 hr
			Left comm. iliac	5 mm	100	120	48 hr
			Right femoral a. occlusion				
573	51	200,000	Left comm. iliac	7 mm	40	60	48 hr
			Left femoral a. occlusion				

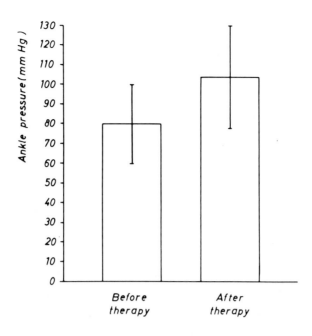

FIGURE 2.   Changes in ankle pressure (ultrasonic Doppler technique) in the course of a 3 day, 30,000 u SK/hr treatment.

REFERENCES

1. **Dotter, C. T., Rosch, J., and Seaman, A. J.,** Selective clot lysis with low dose streptokinase, *Radiology*, 111, 31, 1974.
2. **Duckert, F.,** Contribution to the "Workshop on Streptokinase", AB Kabi, Stockholm, 1974.
3. **Duckert, F., Marbet, G. A., Walter, M., Six, P., Nyman, D., Madar, G., da Silva, M. A., Widmer, L. K., Schmitt, H. E., and Vokal, J.,** Thrombolytic treatment with a streptokinase low dosage regimen, Angiolog. Symp., Engelskirchen, September, 1976.
4. **Gallus, A. S., Hirsh, J., Cade, J. F., Turpie, A. G. G., Walker, I. R., and Gent, M.,** Thrombolysis with a combination of small doses of streptokinase and full doses of heparin, *Semin. Thrombos. Hemost.*, 2, 14, 1975.
5. **Gottlob, R. and Blumel, G.,** Studies on thrombolysis with streptokinase. I. On the penetration of streptokinase into thrombi, *Thrombos. Diathes. haemorrh. (Stuttg.)*, 19, 94, 1968.
6. **Gross, R.,** Blutgerinnung und Fibrinolyse, in *Thrombolyse-Therapie mith Streptokinase. Behring-werke-Mitteilungen,* Elwert, N. G., Ed., Universitats und Verlags-buchhandlung, Marburg/Lahn, 1964, 1.
7. **Latallo, Z. S., Lopaciuk, S., and Meissner, J.,** A combined treatment with Defibrase® and streptokinase, in *Defibrinierung mit Thrombinahnlichen Schlangengiftenzymen,* Martin, M. and Schoop, W., Eds., Verlag Hans Huber, Bern, 1975.
8. **Turpie, A. G. G., Gallus, A. S., Hirsh, J., and Cade, J. F.,** Thrombolysis with a combination of small doses of streptokinase and full dose heparin, 4th Int. Cong. Thrombos. Haemost., Vienna, 1973.

Chapter 12

FOLLOW-UP STUDIES AFTER REMOVAL OF ARTERIAL OCCLUSIONS BY STREPTOKINASE TREATMENT — A 6-YEAR RETROSPECTIVE STUDY*

I. INTRODUCTION

To our knowledge, no more than three studies have been made available up to now concerning continued patency of arteries cleared by lysis. The first two (Martin et al.[2]; Levy et al.[1]) were done by our own group on a relatively small number of patients. The fourth compilation of results (Schulte[3]) includes essential parts of the three above-mentioned studies. On the whole, a surprisingly low tendency for reocclusion of fibrinolytically cleared vessels has been observed.

The present retrospective study followed the fate of 68 arteries where patency had been restored by treatment with streptokinase (Streptase, Behringwerke AG, Marburg/Lahn, West Germany). Attention was focused on the role of both anticoagulant after-treatment and cigarette smoking habit on the reocclusion incident.

II. DESIGN OF THE STUDY

The study covers 67 patients in whom patency of the aorta, the iliac artery, and/or the femoral artery was restored by fibrinolytic treatment at the Aggertalklinik between 1967 and 1974. "Aortic occlusion" should be understood to mean occlusion of the said vessel with or without involvement of one or both common iliac arteries. The statement "removal of an aortic occlusion" was based on the simultaneous patency of the aorta and at least one common iliac artery. The term "removal of an iliac occlusion" comprises the removal of occlusions of either common iliac artery, the external iliac artery, or both the common *and* external iliac arteries. The term "removal of a femoral occlusion" includes the clearance of the popliteal artery, the femoral artery, or both arteries. "Clearing" an artery should be understood to mean restoring complete patency of the arterial section as a result of fibrinolytic treatment, with or without residual stenosis. The mean age of the patients was 56.2 years, the lower age limit was 42 and the upper 78. The case material consisted of 62 males and 5 females. Two different arteries had been cleared fibrinolytically in one patient (the left and right external iliac arteries). Subacute arterial occlusion in chronic arteriopathy was seen 55 times. Vascular occlusions had developed following angiography in three cases, and streptokinase treatment was given in two cases where catheter treatment according to Dotter was unsuccessful. Streptokinase treatment was given for reocclusion after vascular surgery in eight cases.

Occlusions were present in:

- the aorta in 10 cases
- the iliac artery in 36 cases
- the femoral artery in 22 cases

Streptokinase treatment had been preceded by angiography in 50 of the cases. Verification of vascular patency by angiography directly after treatment was possible in

---

* Some paragraphs in this chapter have been prepublished by M. Martin in *Progr. Cardiovasc. Dis.*, 21, 5, 1979. We thank Grune & Stratton for the permission to reprint these items.

37 cases. Clinical methods were employed in diagnosing patency in the remaining ones. With the exception of patients in whom angiography was performed (Patient's Ref. No. 353, 400, 401), the last follow-up investigations were evaluated clinically. Angiographic checkups had been made, however, at intermediate intervals in 11 patients (Patient's Ref. No. 18, 61, 65, 146, 184, 255, 313, 344, 353, 400 and 401).

The *clinical methods* at our disposal were evaluating the arterial pulsation, auscultation, mechanical oscillography at rest and after exercise and measurement of the poststenotic systolic ankle pressure. In two instances (Patient's Ref. No. 61 and 295), the said methods failed to permit safe distinction between patency and possible reocclusion: Ref. No. 61 — a patient in whom a common iliac artery had been cleared earlier by streptokinase treatment, with an appreciable residual stenosis of the ipsilateral external iliac artery and occlusion of a large section of the femoral artery; Ref. No. 292 — a patient in whom the aorta was cleared, with persisting bilateral occlusion of the external iliac artery. Both cases will appear later under the heading of "unexplained vascular status".

Statistical evaluation was initiated in the follow-up trial by separating ten cases of early reocclusions at the hospital for separate consideration. In the remaining 58 occlusions, the vascular status was then evaluated. These cases were divided into three categories:

A.   Cases in which evaluation of the vascular status had been possible.
B.   Patients deceased.
C.   Cases in which evaluation of the vascular status had been impossible for technical reasons ("unexplained vascular status").

Patients had to be included in Category C for various reasons. In two of the cases a definite discrimination between patency or reocclusion was impossible by clinical methods. In two other patients (Ref. No. 207 and 401) the iliac arteries had been cleared by fibrinolysis, and residual stenoses dilated immediately thereafter — surgically in one and by catheter technique in the other. The fate of these two residual stenoses *without* the said secondary treatment must be subject to speculation, and for this reason the cases have been included in Category C (unexplained vascular status). Also included in this category was one patient now living overseas who had not been available for the checkup. Deceased patients were temporarily referred to in Category C, in view of an "obscure" interval existing between the time of the last angiological checkup and the time of death, during which reocclusions might or might not have occurred.

The following reocclusion rates relate·to Category A, exclusively. This appears justified by the fact that any noteworthy difference between the reocclusion rate in Category C (unexplained vascular status) and that in Category A is unlikely. The same applies to Category B (deaths).

III. RESULTS

A. Early Occlusions
Of the 68 arteries cleared, 10 (15%) became blocked again during the patient's stay at the clinic. Table 1 lists the cases, giving locations and precise times of occlusion. In the majority of cases an occlusion occurred in the face of therapeutically effective prothrombin times below 25%.

B. Late Occlusions
1. Reocclusion Rate as a Function of Time
The overall rate of reocclusion showed a steady rise during the first few years after

Table 1
CASES OF EARLY REOCCLUSION SUBDIVIDED ACCORDING TO LOCATION, TIME OF OCCLUSION AND PROTHROMBIN TIME VALUE ON THE DAY OF OCCLUSION

Patient ref. no.	Location	Time of reocclusion (days after ending SK-infusion)	Prothrombin time (%)
82	A. femoralis	2	29
83	A. iliaca	20	65
118	A. femoralis	3	27
143	A. iliaca	15	24
283	A. femoralis	2	33
369	A. femoralis	1	20
472	A. iliaca	2	21
500	A. femoralis	2	25
537	A. femoralis	3	17
554	A. iliaca	4	25

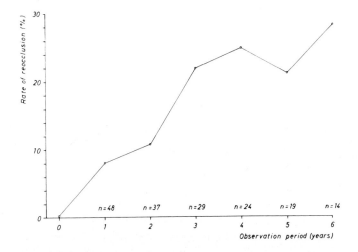

FIGURE 1. Reocclusion rate of the aortae, iliac arteries and femoral arteries during observation period of 6 years.

the end of lysis, and reached 22% at the end of the 3rd year. The incidence then fluctuated between 21 and 29% up to the end of the 6th year (duration of our observation period) (Figure 1; Table 2).

2. Reocclusion Rate as a Function of Location

The *iliac artery*, once cleared by fibrinolysis, showed the least reocclusion tendency (Figure 2), the rate varying between 0 and 12% throughout the 6 year observation. The *femoral artery*, on the other hand, exhibited a continuous rise in the reocclusion rate of up to 50% until the end of the 3rd year, and this level was then maintained up to the 6th year of observation. The reocclusion rate of the lytically cleared *aorta* is presumed to be somewhere between those two extremes, but the relatively small number of cases (n = 8) makes final evaluation difficult (Table 3).

Table 2

DETERMINATION OF RATE OF REOCCLUSION IN RELATION TO THE
TOTAL CASE MATERIAL WITHIN PERIODS OF OBSERVATION OF
BETWEEN 1 AND 6 YEARS

Observation period (years)	Patent	Occluded	% Occluded	Deceased	Unexplained vascular status	Number of patients beyond the observation period	n
1	42	6	8	2	8	0	58
2	33	4	11	2	9	10	58
3	22	6	22	4	7	19	58
4	18	6	25	5	6	23	58
5	15	4	21	5	7	27	58
6	10	4	29	5	4	37	58

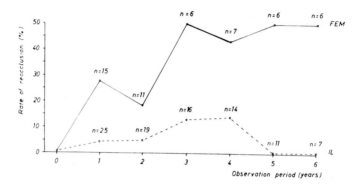

FIGURE 2.   Reocclusion rate listed separately for the iliac and femoral
arteries; n = number of patients.

Table 3

RATE OF REOCCLUSION OF THE
AORTA RENDERED PATENT BY
FIBRINOLYSIS IN DEPENDENCE ON
PERIOD OF OBSERVATION

Observation period (years)	Aorta	
	Patent	Reoccluded
1	7	1
2	6	1
3	4	2
4	2	1
5	1	1
6	0	1

3. Reocclusion Rate as a Function of Cigarette Smoking Habit and Anticoagulant Administration

A spot check was made 3 years after ending lysis for any possible effects of cigarette
smoking or anticoagulant intake on the reocclusion rate. At that time 22 arteries were
patent and 6 were occluded. It was known in each instance whether patients were still
smoking, and whether continuous phenprocouman or acenocoumarol medications
with prothrombin times of between 15 and 25% or Normotest values of between 5 and
15% were carried out. Only patients showing the above values were recorded as anti-

83

Table 4
RATE OF REOCCLUSION 3 YEARS AFTER FIBRINOLYTIC CLEARANCE OF ARTERIES IN THE LOWER EXTREMITIES OF SMOKERS, NONSMOKERS, AND PATIENTS WITH AND WITHOUT THERAPEUTICALLY EFFECTIVE ANTICOAGULANT ADMINISTRATION

Characteristic	Rate of occlusion
Smokers	4/12 (33.4%)
Nonsmokers	2/16 (12.5%)
Anticoagulated	0/8 (0%)
Nonanticoagulated	6/20 (300%)

Note: The difference in reocclusion rate between patients treated with anticoagulants and patients not so treated was statistically significant at p < 0.025.

coagulated. Where medication had been suspended for three months or longer, and/or where the above values were not ensured (as seen from the present and earlier anticoagulation reports), patients were considered "nonanticoagulated".

Patients who had continued smoking after fibrinolytic treatment showed a reocclusion rate of 33.4% vs. 12.5% in patients who had been able to stop smoking (Table 4). The difference was not statistically significant at p < 0.125, thus representing a mere trend. A distinct difference in reocclusion rates of 0 vs. 30% was seen between "anticoagulated" and "nonanticoagulated" patients, which was significant at p < 0.025. Continuous oral anticoagulation thus appears to provide effective prophylaxis following the removal of arterial occlusions. It should be added that all except two of the effectively anticoagulated patients were nonsmokers, and that the anticoagulated population should therefore be looked upon as a combined anticoagulant/nonsmoking group.

IV. SUMMARY

We observed 67 patients, in whom a total of 68 arteries had been made patent by streptokinase treatment, for periods of up to 6 years. In 10 of the 67 cases (= 15%) reocclusion occurred while patients were still in the hospital. The remaining case material with definitely cleared vessels was divided into three groups: (A) patients in whom evaluation of the vascular status was possible; (B) patients who had died in the meantime; and (C) patients in whom the state of the vessels could not be ascertained for technical reasons. Listed below are the results obtained in Group (A):

1. The reocclusion rate showed a steady rise of up to 22% during the first 3 years following streptokinase treatment, and fluctuated around that value up to the end of the 6th year.
2. The iliac artery permitted the best results among the vascular segments cleared. The reocclusion rate was very low, at 0 to 12% throughout the 6 year observation period.
3. The femoral artery reached a reocclusion rate of 50% after 3 years, and this percentage failed to show any appreciable change thereafer.
4. The aortic reocclusion figure was between those ascertained for the iliac and femoral arteries.

5.   Regular and therapeutically effective oral treatment with anticoagulants produced a significant drop in the reocclusion rate. Abstinence from smoking showed a similar trend which did not, however, reach the significance level.

REFERENCES

1. **Levy, H., Schoop, W., Zeitler, E., and Schmidtke, I.,** 4 Jahre Erfahrung mit der thrombolytischen Therapie chronischer Arterienokklusionen. Fruh-und Spatergebnisse bei 350 mit Streptokinase behandelten Verschluβkranken, *Verh. Otsch. Ges. Inn. Med.,* 78, 627, 1972.
2. **Martin, M., Schoop, W., and Zeitler, E.,** *Thrombolyse bei chronischer Arteriopathie,* Hans Huber, Bern, 1970.
3. **Schulte, M.,** Nachuntersuchungen, in *Streptokinase-Therapie bei chronischer arterieller Verschluβkrankheit,* Heinrich, F., Ed., Die Medizinische Verlagsgesellschaft nblt, Marburg/Lahn, 1975.

Chapter 13

OCCURRENCE AND TREATMENT OF BLEEDING ACCIDENTS*

I. INTRODUCTION

The topic of this chapter deals with bleeding accidents in 600 streptokinase treatment series. In 568 cases a maintenance dose of 100,000 u SK/hr was given, in 17 cases: 30,000 u SK/hr, in 10 cases: 5000 u SK/hr, and in 5 cases: escalating amounts of SK. In all, 14 patients were treated over a continuous period of 4 days, 390 patients over a continuous period of 3 days, 128 patients over an uninterrupted period of 2.5 or 2 days, and 11 patients received SK for 1 day or less. Intermittent streptokinase treatment (1st day, SK; 2nd day, SK-heparin; thereafter 12 hr or 24 hr heparin followed by 16 hr or 24 hr SK-heparin) had been used in 57 patients. In 14 patients defibrinogenating measures were substituted for heparin as an anticoagulant principle before, during, and after streptokinase treatment. Tables 1 through 7 show a sequence of major bleeding accidents as they appear from experiences in the streptokinase treatment schemes as shown above.

Bleeding accidents were equally distributed in all streptokinase regimen groups investigated so far. Naturally, because of the greater number of patients included in the continuous 100,000 u SK/hr regimen, most bleedings were reported in this group.

II. OCCURRENCE OF BLEEDING

Gross hematuria was found in 20 patients (3.3%; Table 1). Coagulation values recorded prior to bleeding were — with two exceptions of abnormally lengthened PTT — only moderately changed. According to our experience, no need existed for abruptly terminating treatment. All infusion series were completed as scheduled, but heparin inflow was reduced and hematocrit checks were carried out twice a day.

I.M. bleeding was seen in 16 cases, located in the gluteal muscle 14 times (2.7%; Table 2). As can be seen, I.M. injections were administered up to 4 weeks before start of treatment. Because of unbearable pain, muscular bleeding inevitably led to termination of treatment. Those physicians carrying out fibrinolytic treatments, therefore, urge the hospital staff not to apply I.M. injections in any case.

Bleeding from puncture wounds were recorded in 3 patients (0.5%; Table 3). According to current experiences, they can be avoided if angiography by catheter technique is carried out at least 1 week, and translumbar angiography as well as direct carotid puncture 2 weeks before start of lytic treatment.

Bleeding of the mucous membranes (i.e., conjunctiva, nose, gums; Table 4) were recorded in 21 patients (3.5%) equally distributed over the whole period of treatment. According to our experience, no special measures are required. The oozing mostly ceased by itself. Streptokinase-heparin treatment was never terminated on the grounds of mucosal bleeding. However, if PTT was considerably lengthened, the heparin inflow had to be reduced.

Conceivably, *cerebral accidents* are the one hazard in streptokinase treatment with which physicians are most concerned. As stated before, 600 long-term streptokinase treatment periods were seen, in the course of which 4 patients (0.67%) died — all due to cerebral accidents (Table 5). In two of them, diffuse intracerebral bleeding was proved by autopsy. Yet, because of widespread hemorrhage, no topographic site where

* Parts of this chapter were prepublished by M. Martin in *Rev. Hematol.* We thank PJD Publications Limited for the permission to reprint this material.

Table 1
RECORD OF 20 CASES OF GROSS HEMATURIA IN THE COURSE OF 600 SK-TREATMENT SERIES (3.3%)

Patient ref. no.	Age	Sex	Start of hematuria after onset of infusion (hr)			Measurement of blood coagulation prior to bleeding		
			SK	SK Heparin	Heparin	Prothrombin time (%)	PTT (sec)	Fibrinogen (mg%)
534	64	M	—	48	—	34	67	120
509	51	M	—	48	—	23	79	150
353	65	F	—	48	—	38	81	80
345	56	M	—	—	5	45	90	155
301	59	M	—	—	24	32	70	270
265	39	M	—	—	2	14	90	80
259	59	M	—	—	12	20	77	120
250	69	F	—	12	—	44	109	120
246	58	M	—	—	9	50	87	120
231	51	M	—	—	48	24	153	210
230	53	M	—	24	—	44	72	330
222	48	M	—	—	10	13	68	30
215	42	M	—	29	—	26	65	120
189	58	M	—	—	24	—	—	—
186	59	M	—	—	10	—	—	—
184	50	M	—	—	10	—	—	—
159	57	M	—	48	—	—	—	—
121	58	M	—	48	—	—	—	—
93	58	M	—	—	12	—	—	—
92	56	M	—	12	—	—	—	—
	M = 56					M = 31.4	85.2	146.5

intracerebral bleeding started was definable. Blood clotting values were not strikingly changed prior to bleeding accidents.

The sequence of accidents in relation to the *time* of lytic therapy is worth mentioning. Of the four fatal accidents, two were recorded on the second and two on the third day of treatment. Thus the time factor involved urges us to terminate each streptokinase infusion series as early as possible.

In another 1.3% (n = 8) cerebral episodes — not fully reversible during hospital stay — were recorded (Table 6). Two of these patients underwent angiography, thereby displaying anterior and medial cerebral artery occlusions, respectively. As is evident from these cases, embolic occlusions as cause of cerebral accidents must be taken into consideration.

One minor group (0.83%, n = 5) includes patients suffering from inferior cerebral involvement such as headache, blurred vision, etc. All five patients had recovered completely by the end of hospital stay (Table 7).

III. TREATMENT OF BLEEDING ACCIDENTS

Therapeutic measures in bleeding disorders due to fibrinolytic treatment depended, *inter alia,* on the period of time the infusion had run. Roughly speaking, combined SK-heparin treatment can be divided into three phases (Phases I, II, III — see Chapter 7, Section XIII).

During the first day of treatment *(Phase I),* streptokinase alone was infused.

Phase II of SK-heparin infusion was defined as the period of time when both streptokinase and heparin were infused concomitantly. Phase II lasted from the second day of treatment up to the point when streptokinase infusion was terminated.

Table 2

RECORD OF 16 CASES OF MUSCULAR BLEEDING IN THE COURSE OF 600 SK-TREATMENT SERIES (2.7%)

Patient ref. no.	Age	Sex	Start of muscular bleeding after onset of infusion (hr)		Measurement of blood coagulation prior to bleeding			Bleeding site	Accident prior to bleeding	Time tag between accident and bleeding
			SK	Heparin	Heparin	Prothrombin time (%)	PTT (sec)	Fibrinogen (mg%)			

Patient ref. no.	Age	Sex	SK	Heparin	Heparin	Prothrombin time (%)	PTT (sec)	Fibrinogen (mg%)	Bleeding site	Accident prior to bleeding	Time tag between accident and bleeding
562	59	M	—	48	—	24	142	175	Gluteal m.	I.M. inj.	6 Days
353	65	F	—	48	—	38	81	80	Gluteal m.	I.M. inj.	Unknown
328	62	M	—	8	—	58	34	180	Gluteal m.	I.M. inj.	Unknown
278	60	M	7	—	—	5	—	120	Gluteal m.	I.M. inj.	28 Days
224	61	M	—	36	—	41	103	210	Gluteal m.	I.M. inj.	Unknown
155	46	M	—	36	—	—	—	—	Gluteal m.	I.M. inj.	17 Days
154	56	M	24	—	—	10	—	—	Adductor m.	Sport acc.	2 Days
142	60	M	—	48	—	15	—	—	Gluteal m.	I.M. inj.	15 Days
138	58	M	—	24	—	—	—	—	Gluteal m.	I.M. inj.	14 Days
128	61	M	—	36	—	—	—	—	Gluteal m.	I.M. inj.	6 Days
117	60	F	—	12	—	—	—	—	Gluteal m.	I.M. inj.	13 Days
105	60	M	—	48	—	—	—	—	Gluteal m.	I.M. inj.	Unknown
97	61	M	—	48	—	—	—	—	Gluteal m.	I.M. inj.	Unknown
87	57	M	—	48	—	—	—	—	Tongue		Unknown
64	56	M	24	—	—	—	—	—	Gluteal m.	I.M. inj.	6 Days
61	45	M	24	—	—	—	—	—	Gluteal m.	I.M. inj.	6 Days
	M = 58					M = 27	90	153			M = 11

Note: In most instances an I.M. injection was administered prior to treatment.

Table 3

RECORD OF 3 CASES OF BLEEDING ORIGINATING FROM PUNCTURE WOUNDS IN THE COURSE
OF 600 SK-TREATMENT SERIES (0.5%)

| Patient ref. no. | Age | Sex | Start of bleeding from puncture wound after onset of infusion (hr) | | | Measurement of blood coagulation prior to bleeding | | | Bleeding site | Time lag between arterial puncture and bleeding |
			SK	SK Heparin	Heparin	Prothrombin time (%)	PTT (sec)	Fibrinogen (mg%)		
592	57	F	—	24	—	40	106	105	Femoral a.	6 days
429	58	M	—	28	—	41	86	65	Femoral a.	6 days
42	66	M	—	48	—	—	—	—	Carotid a.	4 days
	M = 60					M = 40.5		96	85	M = 5.3

Table 4

RECORD OF 21 CASES OF MUCOSAL BLEEDING (GINGIVA, CONJUNCTIVA, EAR) IN THE COURSE OF 600 SK-TREATMENT SERIES (3.5%)

Patient ref. no.	Age	Sex	Start of mucosal bleeding after onset of infusion (hr)			Measurement of blood coagulation prior to bleeding		
			SK	SK Heparin	Heparin	Prothrombin time (%)	PTT (sec)	Fibrinogen (mg%)
584	68	M	—	24	—	48	39	160
526	61	M	—	—	6	34	93	120
524	38	M	—	—	12	32	99	290
484	51	M	—	24	—	12	127	370
440	56	M	—	48	—	25	134	230
369	58	M	—	24	—	34	73	40
387	65	M	—	48	—	43	46	90
289	60	M	—	—	12	44	50	120
258	44	F	—	12	—	29	85	80
250	69	F	—	12	—	35	39	160
197	58	M	—	—	24	5	71	120
325	57	M	—	48	—	—	—	—
292	43	M	—	—	36	—	—	—
188	52	M	—	24	—	—	—	—
186	59	M	2	—	—	—	—	—
184	50	M	—	48	—	—	—	—
159	57	M	3	—	—	—	—	—
158	63	M	—	36	—	—	—	—
121	58	M	4	—	—	—	—	—
135	60	M	2	—	—	—	—	—
22	56	M	4	—	—	—	—	—
	M = 56					M = 31	78	162

Phase III covered the period of time following cessation of streptokinase while heparin infusion was maintained.

Basic therapeutic measures in treatment of bleeding disorders are

- Infusion of antiplasmin
- Infusion of antiactivator
- Infusion of fibrinogen
- Infusion of protamine chloride

The application of the above substances depends, *inter alia,* on the period of time the infusions had run (Phase I, II, or III). As mentioned before, appreciable amounts of blood coagulation-inhibiting FDP were found circulating in the bloodstream during the first 24 hr of treatment (Phase I). However, since severe bleeding never occurred during this period of time, no clinical need existed for FDP elimination or neutralization.

After 24 hr from the onset of therapy (i.e., at the beginning of Phase II), a marked depression in fibrinogen was — according to the above data — frequently observed. Bleeding at this time required, therefore, checking of the plasma fibrinogen level and — if necessary — readjustment of fibrinogen up to at least 80 mg%. I.V. infusions of 2 g of fibrinogen were sufficient to arrive at values of this order of magnitude (Figure 1). Since commercial human fibrinogen preparations might be rich in plasminogen generating free circulating plasmin in the SK-contaminated blood, administration of

Table 5

RECORD OF FOUR FATAL CEREBRAL ACCIDENTS IN THE COURSE OF 600 SK-TREATMENT SERIES (0.67%)

Patient ref. no.	Age	Sex	Clinical symptoms	Beginning of symptoms after onset of infusion (hr)			Measurement of blood coagulation prior to clinical symptoms		
				SK	SK Heparin	Heparin	Prothrombin time (%)	PTT (sec)	Fibrinogen (mg%)
577	60	M	Loss of consciousness (diffuse cerebral bleeding)	—	20	—	42	82	240
567	38	M	Progressively increasing clouding of consciousness (subdural bleeding)	—	7	—	39	36	240
414	72	M	Progressively increasing clouding of consciousness (stroke)	—	32	—	54	65	50
305	64	M	Loss of consciousness	—	48	—	34	38	120
	M = 59						M = 42	55	163

Table 6

RECORD OF EIGHT CEREBRAL ACCIDENTS WHICH WERE NONREVERSIBLE DURING HOSPITAL STAY IN THE COURSE OF 600 SK-TREATMENT SERIES (1.3%)

Patient ref. no.	Age	Sex	Clinical symptoms	Beginning of symptoms after onset of infusion (hr)			Measurement of blood coagulation prior to clinical symptoms		
				SK	SK Heparin	Heparin	Prothrombin time (%)	PTT (sec)	Fibrinogen (mg%)
494	48	M	Double vision	—	12	—	30	45	88
317	61	M	Subdural hematoma (clinically evident 24 days after lytic therapy)	—	—	—	—	—	—
282	44	M	Paralysis of abducens nerve, subarachnoidal bleeding	—	9	—	30	51	120
262	63	M	Hemiamaurosis	—	—	1	26	107	i20
247	56	M	Aphasia	—	—	1	37	125	180
171	78	M	Cerebral embolism	—	2	—	—	(PTZ 31 sec)	180
95	63	M	Cerebral embolism	—	—	24	—	—	—
D404	43	M	Clouding of consciousness, sensorial aphasia	—	—	1 ½ (Defibrase)	0	>300	60
	M = 59						M = 31	82	138

Table 7

RECORD OF FIVE CEREBRAL ACCIDENTS WHICH WERE REVERSIBLE DURING
HOSPITAL STAY IN THE COURSE OF 600 SK-TREATMENT SERIES (0.83%)

Ref. no.	Age	Sex	Clinical symptoms	Beginning of symptoms after onset of infusion (hr)			Measurement of blood congulation prior to clinical symptoms		
				SK	SK Heparin	Heparin	Prothrombin time (%)	PTT (sec)	Fibrinogen (mg%)
517	52	M	Headache, blurred vision	—	5	—	26.5	55	80
469	37	M	Headache	—	3½	—	47	41	120
289	60	M	Headache	—	—	36	44	50	120
333	58	M	Transitory paralysis of the right occulomotorius nerve	—	48	—	42	104	120
204	53	M	Headache, vomiting, stiffness of the neck	21	—	—	—	—	—
	M = 52						M = 40	63	110

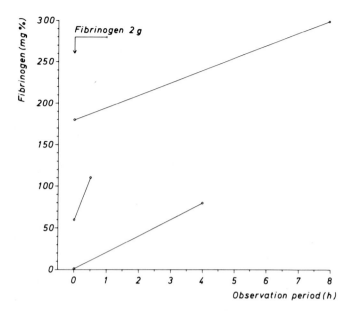

FIGURE 1. Increase in plasma fibrinogen concentration after I.V. administration of 2 g human fibrinogen in 13 patients after terminating SK treatment. The fibrinogen amount applied was, on the average, sufficient for elevating the fibrinogen concentration by 100 mg%.

antiactivators such as trans-AMCHA and antiplasmins such as Trasylol® should precede each fibrinogen infusion. For fibrinogen restitution, KABI-fibrinogen was given preference, since the latter was shown to contain plasminogen in a very low concentration,[10] namely, 0.03 Remmert and Cohen u/mℓ of a 355 mg% fibrinogen solution (= 2.7% of normal) (Table 8).

The drug of choice for inhibiting plasminemia following fibrinogen infusion is Trasylol®. Trasylol® is a polypeptide of mol wt 6200 isolated from parotid gland and lung tissues. Its action on plasmin is uncompetitive. To a lesser degree, plasminogen activation by streptokinase is inhibited competitively.[5]

Plasmin activities following addition of 500 u streptokinase to 1 mℓ each of normal plasma and euglobulin were fully inhibited by 60 u Trasylol®/mℓ (Figure 2). This finding is in agreement with similar results of Amris.[1] Furthermore, inhibiting effects were tested on plasma samples of patients undergoing streptokinase treatment. As diagramed in Figure 3, plasmin concentrations in the early period of streptokinase infusion were readily neutralized by 8 u Trasylol®/mℓ. As human plasma volume averages 2500 mℓ, 20,000 u Trasylol® might, therefore, be sufficient for plasmin inhibiting treatment. However, Trasylol® displayed a very short half-life of only 10 min during the first ½ hr and of 150 min later on,[2] and, therefore, a tenfold Trasylol® injection of 200,000 u is recommended in case of urgent streptokinase treatment discontinuation and fibrinogen replacement. This Trasylol® dose can be regarded as a reliable safeguard against plasminemia generated in the course of fibrinogen readjustment.

The active isomer of synthetic aminomethylcyclohexane carboxylic acid (trans-AMCHA) has been shown to be a competitive inhibitor of plasmin activation by streptokinase and, at much higher concentrations, an uncompetitive inhibitor of plasmin.[3] According to our experience, trans-AMCHA can be regarded as an antifibrinolytic principle much less powerful than Trasylol®. Activator strength in the plasma of patients under conventional SK treatment was tested on a clot lysis assay consisting of bovine plasminogen and fibrin. Increasing admixture of trans-AMCHA concentrations

Table 8
PLASMINOGEN CONTENT OF
VARIOUS FIBRINOGEN
PREPARATIONS

**Plasminogen concentration per
355 mg% fibrinogen**

Human plasma	100 % =	1.2	Remmert & Cohen u/m*l*
Fibrinogen (Immuno)	134 % =	1.6	Remmert & Cohen u/m*l*
Fibrinogen (Behringwerke)	13.7 % =	0.16	Remmert & Cohen u/m*l*
Fibrinogen (Deutsche Kabi)	2.7 % =	0.03	Remmert & Cohen u/m*l*

Note: All plasminogen values were calculated on the basis of a 335 mg% fibrinogen concentration (normal value of plasma).

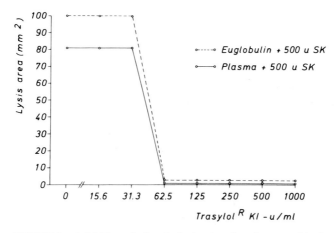

FIGURE 2.　Inhibition of plasmin in 1 m*l* native plasma and in 1 m*l* euglobulin derived from 1 m*l* plasma. Activation was accomplished by adding 500 u SK to each of the samples. Inhibition was recorded after adding rising amounts of Trasylol®. Complete inhibition was seen when the Trasylol® concentration exceeded 63 u/m*l*.

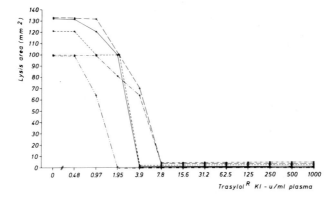

FIGURE 3.　Inhibition of plasmin in 1 m*l* plasma drawn from patients during the first 2 hr of streptokinase treatment. Complete inhibition resulted after addition of 8 u Trasylol®.

Table 9
PRELIMINARY PROPOSAL FOR EMERGENCY TREATMENT IN BLEEDING ACCIDENTS UNDER FIBRINOLYTIC THERAPY USING A STANDARDIZED STREPTOKINASE INFUSION SCHEME

Components related to hemostatic defects	First day of treatment (SK-infusion 100000 u/hr)	Second and third day of treatment (SK-heparin infusion 100000 u SK · 1500 u hep/hr)	Fourth day of treatment (heparin infusion 500—1500 u/hr
Circulating SK	No therapeutic measures necessary (no bleeding accidents expected)	Discontinuation of infusion (SK <0.5 u/mℓ after 1 hr)	No treatment (no SK circulating)
Circulating plasmin		Trans-AMCHA 2g q 2 hr Trasylol® 200000 u q 2 hr	No treatment (no plasmin circulating)
Circulating FDP		No treatment (only minute amounts of FDP circulating)	No treatment (no FDP circulating)
Circulating heparin		Discontinuation of infusion; protamine 1% 5 mℓ	Discontinuation of infusion;
Low fibrinogen		Trosyiol® 200,000 u; fibrinogen 2 g	protamine 1% 5mℓ No treatment (fibrinogen >70 mg%)

resulted in falling activator activity. However, full inhibition was not achieved until 10 mg trans-AMCHA was added to 1 mℓ plasma, i.e., 25 g/2500 mℓ plasma[9]. Conceivably, these drug quantities equaling ¼ of the DL50 are impossible to administer. Furthermore, a relatively short half-life of 15 min during the first ½ hr and of 2 hr thereafter[7] will additionally weaken the antifibrinolytic effect. In conclusion, we might say that trans-AMCHA administration can be looked upon as a possible adjunct to, but not likely as a reliable substitute for, Trasylol®.

Overdosage of heparin during Phases II and III of lytic treatment is signaled by prolongation of the partial prothrombin time beyond the 100 sec mark (i.e., a PTT above 2½ times normal). Adequate measures are I.V. administration of 10 mℓ 1% protamine chloride, which leads to immediate normalization of blood coagulation.

IV. SUMMARY

Therapeutic actions in bleeding accidents during streptokinase treatment depend on the period of time the infusion has run. During Phase I of streptokinase-heparin treatment (i.e., in the first 24 hr period where streptokinase alone was administered) no therapeutic measures are proposed since — according to our experience — no accidents of importance are to be expected (Table 9). Phase II of streptokinase treatment is featured by combined streptokinase-heparin infusion, resulting in relatively low but stable plasma fibrinogen concentrations. Emergency measures are consistent with restoring fibrinogen. Prior to fibrinogen infusion, antifibrinolytic agents should be administered to avoid marked plasminemia via activation of fibrinogen-bound plasminogen. A dose of 200,000 u Trasylol®/mℓ plasma will eliminate plasmin activities for at least 1 hr. Reliable antistreptokinase preparations designed for clinical purposes are not available for the time being, and immediate streptokinase elimination from the organism is therefore impossible. However, as the half-life of streptokinase is very brief, averaging 20 min, it is, as a rule, sufficient to discontinue the infusion, whereupon only minimal streptokinase activity in the blood will be found after a period of 1½ hr.

REFERENCES

1. **Ambris, C. J.**, Inhibition of fibrinolytic and thromboplastic activity by Trasylol, *Scand. J. Haemat.*, 3, 19, 1966.
2. **Beller, F. K., Epstein, M. D., and Kaller, H.**, Distribution, half-life time and placental transfer of the protease inhibitor trasylol, *Thrombos. Diathes. Haemorrh. (Stuttg.)*, 16, 302, 16.
3. **Dubber, A. H. C., McNicol, G. P., Douglas, A. S.**, Amino methyl cyclohexane carboxylic acid (AMCHA) — a new synthetic fibrinolytic inhibitor, *Br. J. Haemat.*, 11, 237, 1965.
4. **Dubber, A. H. C., McNicol, G. P., Douglas, A. S., and Melander, B.**, Some properties of the antifibrinolytically active isomer of aminomethylcyclohexane carboxylic acid, *Lancet*, II, 1317, 1964.
5. **Dubber, A. H. C., McNicol, G. P., Uttley, D., and Douglas, A. S.**, In vitro and in vivo studies with Trasylol, an anticoagulant and a fibrinolytic inhibitor, *Br. J. Haemat.*, 14, 31, 1968.
6. **Fischer, M.**, Vergleichende Untersuchungen der Fibrinolyse-inhibitoren AMCHA, EACA und PAMBA, *Wien. Zxchr. Inn. Med.*, 47, 143, 1966.
7. **Kaller, H.**, Enterale Resorption und Elimination von 4-Aminomethylcyclohexancarbonsäure (AMCHA) und Aminocapronsäure (ACS) beim Menschen, *Nauyn-Schmiedebergs Arch. Pharmak. Exp. Pathol.*, 256, 160, 1967.
8. **Marx, R., Clemente, P., Werle, E., and Appel, W.**, Zum Problem eines Anticlotes in der internen Thrombotherapie mit Fibrinolytica, *Blut*, 5, 367, 1959.
9. **Martin, M.**, *Treatment of Bleeding Accidents During Fibrinolytic Therapy*, Vol. 1, PJD Publ. Ltd., Westbury, N.Y., 1980.
10. **Auel, H. and Martin, M.**, Plasminogengehalt in Humanfibrogen-Praparationen verschiedener Hersteller, *J. Clin. Chem. Clin. Biochem.*, 15, 397, 1977.

Chapter 14

OTHER SIDE EFFECTS, EXCEPT BLEEDING*

I. FEVER

Fever was a frequently recorded side effect while infusing streptokinase. According to current experience, about 22% of all patients undergoing streptokinase treatment showed temperatures above 38°C. Temperatures during streptokinase therapy displayed a pattern of infrequency and unpredictability, but responded promptly to 1 g Novalgin® I.V. (sodium phenyl-dimethyl-pyrazolone-methyl-aminomethane sulfonate = sodium metamizol, Hoechst AG, Frankfurt/M., West Germany). Very early in this study Novalgin 1 g I.V. was regularly administered as a prophylactic measure just before nighttime. This relatively simple measure turned out to be a reliable safeguard against unforeseeable rises in temperature.

II. LOWERED RESISTANCE

Upon terminating streptokinase treatment, a limited number of patients felt tired and weak for about 1 week, as if they had just recovered from the flu. One case of bronchial pneumonia, one case of abacterial meningitis, and two cases of sepsis several days after ending infusion point to a state of lowered resistance after conclusion of streptokinase treatment. Patients regarded "at risk" for imminent infection were put on broad-spectrum antibiotics (e.g., ampicillin, cephalosporins).

III. ALLERGIC SKIN MANIFESTATIONS

Within 3 to 6 days after ending streptokinase treatment, characteristic skin manifestations resembling eruptions similar to those seen in the Schönlein-Henoch syndrome were recorded in 5 patients. The symptoms consisted of a hemorrhagic purpura of the lower leg skin, as well as swelling and pain in both knee and ankle joints. The above signs subsided promptly within 1 to 2 weeks and had no aftereffects whatsoever. Since coumarol medication was regularly given during that period of time, no definite answer can be given to the question as to how far a direct coumarol-linked vessel wall damage, as described by Stefanelli et al.[15] might be involved.

IV. ACCELERATED ERYTHROCYTE SEDIMENTATION RATE (ESR)

During streptokinase treatment, ESRs went through a sequence of typical alterations. At the beginning of streptokinase treatment a sharp ESR slow down and after cessation of therapy an abnormal ESR acceleration were recorded. Under streptokinase infusion, the mean ESR remained slow (averaging 3/9 mm according to Westergren). By contrast, a few days after terminating streptokinase treatment, the ESR accelerated sharply up to values around 60/90 mm on the 8th posttreatment day. Later on, ESRs tended to normalize again (Figure 1). From this it becomes evident that postlytic ESR acceleration is a laboratory side effect by no means related to a secondary illness.

Up to now, no explanation for the phenomenon of reduction in sedimentation after

---

* Parts of this chapter were prepublished by M. Martin in *Rev. Hematol.* We thank PJD Publications Limited for the permission to reprint this material.

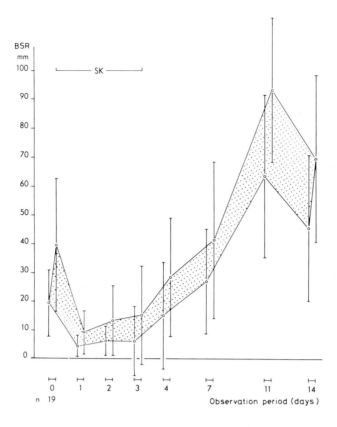

FIGURE 1. Erythrocyte sedimentation rate (ESR) according to
Westergren prior to, during, and after streptokinase treatment. After
a slowing down of ESR *during* therapy, a continuous acceleration of
BSR *after* therapy, reaching a peak on the 11th day after start of
treatment, was recorded. Brackets = standard deviation; dotted area
= values between the 1 hr and 2 hr recording.

streptokinase treatment can be established. However, the parallelism between the fall
in fibrinogen and retardation of ESR at the beginning of treatment would suggest a
link between these two findings. Further, the noticeable timing between acceleration
of ESR and allergic reactions 1 to 2 weeks after ending streptokinase treatment would
point also to a link between these two phenomena.

V. CHANGES IN SERUM ENZYME PATTERNS

Continuous monitoring of GOT, GPT, and alkaline phosphatase (AP) gave evidence
of a significant rise in these three enzymes (Figure 2) during the course of streptokinase
treatment. Before treatment, average GOT, GPT, and AP concentrations were measured at 10.6, 7.8 and 43 mV/ml, respectively. One day after conclusion of streptokinase treatment, the values had amounted to figures as high as 35 (3.3 × normal), 43
(5.5 × normal), and 79 (1.8 × normal) mV/ml respectively. Thereafter, a decrease in
the enzyme concentrations was recorded, leveling off to normal after a period of 14
days.[13]

These changes in the pattern of serum enzymes under the influence of streptokinase
were confirmed by Schmidt et al.[14] in 1972. Additionally, the same authors investigated
the behavior of GLDH (mitochondrial glutamate dehydrogenase, index of severe cel-

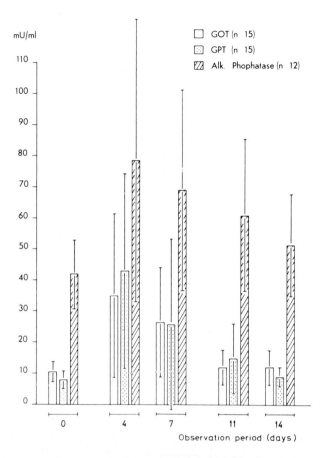

FIGURE 2. Pattern showing rises in serum enzymes immediately
after conclusion of streptokinase treatment.

lular damage), GGTP (γ-glutamyl transpeptidase, evaluating cholestasis), CHE (cho-
linesterase, index of the capacity of protein synthesis in the liver), LDH (lactic dehydrogenase), and CPK (creatin phosphatase kinase, indexes of possible involvement of
red blood cells and skeletal muscle) under lytic treatment. During streptokinase infusion GOT, GPT, GGTP, GLDH, and AP showed a significant rise, while CHE fell
well below the pretreatment concentration. Furthermore, an enhanced Bromsulphalein
retention in the plasma was demonstrated. According to Schmidt et al.,[14] the above
changes are indicative of both a disturbance of hepatic cellular/subcellular membrane
permeability and an intrahepatic cholestasis. Moreover, the authors were able to show
by animal experiments that the change in the enzymatic patterns were not due to the
action of streptokinase itself, but exclusively to plasminemia accompanying beginning
and end of fibrolytic therapy.

Interestingly, creatin phosphatase kinase (CPK) concentrations originating from
damaged skeletal and heart muscles were not affected by lytic therapy, thus enabling
the physician to make use of CPK measurement for the assessment of myocardial
infarction immediately after conclusion of streptokinase therapy.

VI. NEW ARTERIAL OBSTRUCTIONS IN CONNECTION WITH STREPTOKINASE TREATMENT

It was a momentous experience when we learned that not only thrombus dissolution
but also newly formed occlusions were recorded after streptokinase treatment.[3]

Table 1

**NEW OBSTRUCTIONS OCCURRING AT
UNKNOWN TIME IN CONNECTION
WITH STREPTOKINASE TREATMENT**

Patient ref. no.	Location	Comment
5	Femoral artery	—
6	Femoral artery	—
103	Common iliac artery	2 Stenoses: 1 widened and 1 deteriorated

The incidence of both thrombus dissolution and formation of new thrombus material during the same treatment period is shown in Figure A-34 to A-36 in the Appendix.

In the meantime, several groups have reported on acute arterial occlusions connected with streptokinase treatment (Hume et al.[1]: 5 cases; Verstraete et al.[2]: 1 case; Heinrich et al.[11]: 1 case; Ehringer et al.[12]: 3 cases).

There is great practical interest concerning the question as to when a fresh arterial occlusion might be formed. Thoretically, new occlusions or further aggravation of stenoses could develop

- Between first angiography and SK infusion
- During therapy
- After terminating therapy (prior to or after the angiographic checkup)

A. New Obstructions Formed at Unknown Point in Time

Of 17 new obstructions, 3 were formed sometime between the pretreatment and checkup angiographies, it being impossible to fix the exact time (Table 1). All newly occluded stenoses in this group were extremely narrow, to the extent that their occlusion was neither perceived by the patient, nor traced in the oscillogram or in the values of ultrasonic pressure measurement. It cannot be ruled out with certainty that one or more of these freshly formed occlusions had settled immediately after the first angiographic procedure and, therefore, had nothing to do with subsequent lytic treatment.

B. New Obstructions Formed During Streptokinase Infusion

New occlusions observed during streptokinase infusion comprised, *inter alia*, microembolic events. Microemboli frequently chipped off from thrombi undergoing lytic disintegration and could be looked upon, in a certain sense, as first indication of successful clot removal. Principal signs of embolization were pain, as well as transient cyanotic discoloration of a toe or some other small and circumscribed tissue region.

In one patient, microemboli were swept into peripheral renal arteries, the source being a renal artery stenosis of crumbly and irregular type (Table 2).

In a second patient, a left iliac occlusion was removed by 3 day streptokinase treatment. At the time of clearance, am embolic femoral occlusion in the same limb was recorded.

A similar incident developed during a streptokinase treatment of a chronic iliac stenosis. After 1 day streptokinase treatment, the iliac narrowing widened, but during that period a fresh femoral occlusion on the same side was recorded. In contrast to the foregoing case, this new and probably embolic occlusion was again removed by further SK-heparin treatment.

We feel that supplementary heparin infusion to streptokinase might be a reliable tool to prevent further apposition of thrombus material around embolic masses. As

Table 2
NEW OBSTRUCTIONS OCCURRING DURING THE COURSE OF
STREPTEKINASE TREATMENT

Patient ref. no.	Location	Time of occlusion (days after starting infusion)	Comment
26	Femoral a.	1	Widening of a left iliac stenosis. At the same time, occurrence of a left femoral occlusion on the same side. Restoration of patency 2 days later.
50	Renal a.	0.5	Aggravation of a renal artery stenosis. Embolization into branches of the renal artery.
415	Femoral a.	3	Removal of an iliac occlusion on the left side. At the same time, new occlusion of the left femoral artery.

plasminogen averages 0.5% under conventional SK dosage regimen, new therapeutic appositions would be extremely poor in plasminogen and scarcely amenable to lysis by further streptokinase infusion.

C. New Obstructions After Ending Streptokinase Infusion

Eleven new occlusions or aggravations of stenoses were recorded during the first week after conclusion of streptokinase therapy (Table 3). In one of these patients, a femoral occlusion developed 10 hr after the breakdown of an infusion pump (since then, a time marker was taped to the syringe and the nurse on duty urged to check the device every second hour, day and night). In another female patient, treated for a left iliac occlusion and a right iliac stenosis, a newly formed aortic occlusion set in 4 days after ending infusion. There was no anticoagulant treatment during that time (Figure A-35, Appendix). Immediately after the checkup angiography, the thrombotic masses were removed by vascular surgery.

One patient displayed an aggravation of an internal carotid stenosis, with subsequent embolic occlusion of the ipsilateral medial cerebral artery half a day after ending streptokinase infusion, but under subsequent heparin administration.

In the remaining group, 1 myocardial infarction and occlusions of 1 aortic, 3 iliac and 2 femoral stenoses, and 2 embolic occlusions of calf arteries were recorded.

Regarding the origin of newly formed vascular occlusions, only hypotheses can be brought forward. Basically, the formation of new occlusions or deterioration of stenoses after streptokinase therapy can be explained by

- Embolism
- Thrombus formation *in loco*
- Intimal swelling due to allergic reactions
- General hypercoagulatability

Two examples of *embolization* into calf arteries were mentioned in the foregoing paragraph. *Newly formed thrombi* may develop on the intimal surface by means of a direct contact between blood and subendothelial collagen fibers,[7-9] the latter being exposed after lytic removal of old thrombotic coating. The fact that occlusions settled at the same time when soaring anti-SK titers, accelerated erythrocyte sedimentation rates, skin manifestations, and joint swellings occurred also points to an underlying *hyperergic mechanism.*

Occlusion of small and medium sized arteries, accompanied by cutaneous exanthem and joint swelling 1 to 2 weeks after withdrawal of the antigen, were documented in a

Table 3
NEW OBSTRUCTIONS DEVELOPING AFTER ENDING STREPTOKINASE INFUSION

Patient ref. no.	Location	Time of occlusion (days after ending SK infusion)	Prothrombin time (%) on day of occlusion	Comments
87	External iliac artery	2	100	No anticoagulants
95	Internal carotid artery	0.5	—	Stenosis aggravated during heparin infusion, cerebral embolization
100	Aorta + common iliac artery	4	100	No anticoagulants
103	Femoral artery	Within 1st week	100	No anticoagulants
131	Common iliac artery	5	100	Anticoagulants discontinued
147	Femoral artery	10 hr	—	Infusion machine broke down
192	Posterior tibial artery	1	6.8	Probably embolic originating from aortic stenosis
197	Posterior tibial artery	1	13	Embolic, probably originating from iliac stenosis
307	Femoral artery	3	35	—
365	Coronary artery	4	25	Myocardial infarction
447	Iliac artery	4	18	—

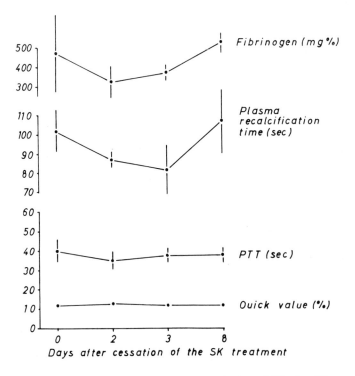

FIGURE 3.   Fibrinogen level (1), whole blood recalcification (2), partial thromboplastin time (3) and prothrombin time (4) prior to, and 2, 3 and 8 days after ending streptokinase administration. Means and standard deviations for 6 patients.

number of publications dealing with allergic side effects of another strong antigen, namely, penicillin.[4-6]

Hypercoagulability was recorded in 6 patients without any further anticoagulating measures after cessation of streptokinase treatment (Figure 3). A marked reduction in the whole blood recalcification time and a slight fall in partial thromboplastin time were measured 2 and 3 days after ending streptokinase therapy. Of these 6 patients, nonanticoagulated after streptokinase treatment, 3 developed acute arterial occlusions, thus indicating a need for anticoagulant measures at least during the 1st week of lytic treatment.

Obviously, if a fresh occlusion sets in after streptokinase treatment, it is very difficult, if not impossible, to isolate one single cause for this incident. As was pointed out by Duckert and Streuli,[10] the induction of thrombosis is an extremely complex process, involving a great number of still unknown factors.

REFERENCES

1. **Hume, M., Gurewich, V., Dealy, J. B., and Gajewski, J.**, Streptokinase for chronic arterial disease; effective lysis and thromboembolic complications, in *Thrombolytic Therapy*, Mammen, E. F., Anderson, G. F., and Barnhart, M. I., Eds., F. K. Schattauer-Verlag, Stuttgart, 1971, 229.
2. **Verstraete, M., Vermylen, J., and Donati, M. B.**, The effect of streptokinase infusion on chronic arterial occlusions and stenoses, *Ann. Int. Med.*, 74, 377, 1971.
3. **Martin, M., Schoop, W., and Zeitler, E.**, Frische arterielle Verschlüsse als Komplikation der Infusions behandlung mit Streptokinase, *Dtsch. Med. Wochenschr.*, 94, 1240, 1969.
4. **Martin, M., Schulte, P., Sobbe, A., Klammer, H. L., Schulz, D., and Raschke, E.**, Multiple Verschlüsse grosserer Arterien nach Penicillin-Gabe, *Dtsch. Med. Wochenschr.*, 98, 1333, 1973.
5. **Sunder-Plassmann, P.**, Klinische Beobachtungen zur Frage der Penicillin-Allergie, *Langenbeck's Arch. Klin. Chür.*, 316, 359, 1966.
6. **Sunder-Plassmann, P., Isfort, A., Esch, R., and Forck, G.**, Pathogenese und Therapie akuter Arterienverschlüsse, *Med. Klin.*, 62, 87, 1967.
7. **Niewiarowski, S., Bankowski, E., and Rogowicka, I.**, Studies on the adsorption and activation of the Hageman-Factor (Factor XII) by collagen and elastin, *Thrombos. Diathes. Haemorrh. (Stuttg.)*, 14, 387, 1965.
8. **Martin, M. and Staubesand, J.**, Intravasale Thrombusbildung durch elektrischen Strom und Thrombolyse; eine elektroenmikroskopische Studie, *Thrombos. Diathes. Haemorrh. (Stuttg.)*, 18, 570, 1967.
9. **Ashford, T. P. and Freiman, D. G.**, The role of endothelium in the initial phases of thrombosis, *Am. J. Pathol.*, 50, 257, 1967.
10. **Duckert, F. and Streuli, F.**, Role of coagulation in thrombosis, in *Pathogenesis and Treatment of Thromboembolic Diseases*, Koller, F., Duckert, F., and Streuli, F., Eds., F. K. Schattauer-Verlag, Stuttgart, 1966, 185.
11. **Heinrich, F., Schmutzler, R., and Braun, H.**, Die medikamentöse Eroffnung chronischer Gliedmaßenarterienverschlüsse, *Therapiewoche*, 21, 1317, 1971.
12. **Ehringer, H., Fischer, M., Lechner, K., and Mayrhofer, E.**, Thrombolytische Therapie nich akuter arterieller Verschlüsse, *Dtsch. Med. Wochenschr.*, 95, 610, 1970.
13. **Martin, M., Schoop, W., and Zeitler, E.**, *Thrombolyse bei chronischer Arteriopathie*, Verlag Hans Huber, Bern, 1970.
14. **Schmidt, E., Poliwoda, H., Buhl, V., Alexander, K., and Schmidt, F. W.**, Observations of enzyme elevations in the serum during streptokinase treatment, *J. Clin. Pathol.*, 25, 650, 1972.
15. **Stefanelli, N., Tulzer, H., and Wewelka, F.**, Hautnekrosen als Nebenwirkung der Therapie mit Antikoagulantien. *Thrombos. Diathes. Haemorrh. (Stuttg.)*, 5, 136, 1960.

Chapter 15

GENERAL ASSESSMENT AND DISCUSSION OF LYTIC RESULTS IN CHRONIC ARTERIAL OCCLUSIONS AND STENOSES*

Nonorganized thrombotic masses located in the iliac arteries and the aorta were described by Jäger[9] in his fundamental autopsy reports on four individuals suffering from severe chronic arterial occlusions. Similar observations were published by Klostermeyer.[10] Mittelmeier[11] held that thrombus organization might be hampered or even blocked, if clots were adherent to arterial walls affected by marked sclerosis: "During the course of time, thrombotic material (in sclerotic arteries) decays to crumbly, pasty, initially brownish, but later yellowish glossy masses. The same is true of thrombi located in large elastic vessels, even if sclerosis had not developed to such an extent".

In the early 1960s Rosolleck[12,13] was the first to tackle the problem on how far chronic arterial occlusion masses might respond to streptokinase treatment. The result of his experiments dealing with longstanding arterial thrombi derived from amputated limbs provided evidence that, on principle, a dissolution of old intravascular thrombi was possible.

Gottlob and co-workers[7,8] worked up this subject more extensively, thereby fully confirming the above observation. Furthermore, the results of this group even suggested that relatively old thrombi might respond better to streptokinase incubation than younger ones.

Independently, five papers were published in 1968[1-5] dealing with clinical results of streptokinase treatment of chronic arterial occlusions and stenoses (Table 1). Their findings indicated that, in general, longstanding arterial obstructions could be removed by streptokinase treatment. Later on, further contributions corroborated the above findings and went into more detail.[14-16,24,26]

Surveying the outcome of the present study devoted to streptokinase treatment of chronic arterial occlusions of the lower limbs, we found that a clearance rate of around 75% could be achieved if femoral and iliac occlusions were treated within the first 2 weeks after onset of symptoms. A significantly reduced clearance rate down to 57% had to be anticipated in femoral and iliac occlusions of 2 to 6 weeks standing. Femoral arteries were virtually nonlysable after 3 months, and iliac occlusions after 6 months of age.

These retrospective results clearly call for an immediate diagnosis and instantaneous start of streptokinase infusion after the patient's admission to the hospital. Because best therapeutic results could be achieved during the first 2 weeks following the occlusion incident, we are cautious about the question as to what extent angiography should be performed prior to treatment. According to current experience, about 1 week has to pass after angiography before lytic treatment can start without the risk of bleeding from the puncture wound. Thus, valuable time would be lost and therapeutic results jeopardized. However, angiography is useful, especially in cases where the occlusion period remains difficult to ascertain by the patient's account and where some morphological clues on the occlusion age would be helpful.

By contrast, the outcome of lytic therapy on chronic arterial *stenoses* could *only* be predicted by estimating its morphologic shape in the angiogram. Compared with this, the stenosis age was not a dominant factor for predicting the therapeutic outcome of lytic treatment. Narrowings of short, irregular, and crumbly shapes, as summarized

* Some paragraphs in this chapter have been prepublished by M. Martin in *Progr. Cardiovasc. Dis.*, 21, 5, 1979. We thank Grune & Stratton for the permission to reprint these items.

Table 1

ACCUMULATION OF REPORTS DEALING WITH REMOVAL OF CHRONIC
ARTERIAL OCCLUSIONS AND WIDENING OF STENOSES

	Type of obstruction						
	Femoral		Iliac		Aortic		
Author	St[a]	Oc[b]	St	Oc	St	Oc	Therapeutic results and comments
Alexander et al.[1]	2	23	5	5	—	—	Removal of 4 femoral occlusions 5 wk—9 mo of age Removal of 2 iliac occlusions 5 wk—6 wk of age
Ehringer and Fischer[2]	—	8	—	1	—	—	Removal of 5 femoral occlusions 5 day—5 wk of age
Heinrich and Schmutzler[16]	6	22	—	31	2	6	Removal of 8 femoral occlusions less than 8 wk of age Widening of 3 femoral stenoses less than 2 yr of age Removal of 3 iliac occlusions less than 1 yr of age Widening of 13 iliac stenoses less than 2 yr of age Removal of 1 aortic occlusion
Kaindl et al.[3]	—	10	—	1	—	—	No success. Occlusions between 5—15 mo of age
Verstraete et al.[25]	5	17	16	11	1	2	Only 4 occlusions less than 2 mo old Removal of 1 femoral artery 21 day of age Removal of 1 iliac artery (common femoral artery) 4 mo of age Removal of 1 aortic occlusion 1 yr of age
Le Veen and Diaz[14]	—	26	—	3	—	1	Removal of 10 femoral occls. 6 hr—9 mo of age Removal of 1 iliac occlusion 14 day of age
Deutsch and Ehringer[24]	—	53	—	13	—	—	Removal of 14 femoral occlusions 6 day—6 wk of age Removal of 2 femoral occlusions 6 wk—6 mo of age Removal of 7 iliac occlusions 6 day—6 wk of age Removal of 2 iliac occlusions 6 wk—6 mo of age
Schoop et al.[4]	—	34	—	43	—	7	Removal of 1 femoral occlusion 10 mo of age Removal of 7 iliac occlusions 5 wk—4 yr of age Removal of 3 aortic occlusions 6 mo—7 yr of age
Schoop et al.[5]	11	—	5	—	1	—	Widening of 3 femoral stenoses Widening of 5 iliac stenoses Widening of 1 aortic stenosis
Martin et al.[26]	25	98	73	97	4	15	Removal of 4 femoral occlusions Removal of 16 iliac occlusions Removal of 4 aortic occlusions Widening of 5 femoral stenoses Widening of 42 iliac stenoses Widening of 3 aortic stenoses
Persson et al.[15]	—	14	—	4	—	—	Therapeutic failure in 8 femoral and 1 iliac occlusion of several mo or yr standing. Clearance in 6 femoral and 3 iliac occlusions below 10 days of age

[a]   St = Stenosis
[b]   Oc = Occlusion

in Chapter 10, were best suited for streptokinase therapy. This significance of morphological criteria makes angiography a necessary prerequisite for lytic treatment of arterial narrowings.

Chronic arterial obstructions located in the upper half of the body, such as narrowings (four cases) and occlusions (four cases) of the internal carotid artery, as well as occlusions of the brachiocephalic truncus (two cases), did not respond to streptokinase treatment and might possibly be regarded as unsuitable targets for lytic therapy.

One point that deserves broader discussion concerns the question as to how far clinical trials investigating the clearance rate of arterial occlusions or the widening of chronic stenoses, as done in this study, can be properly conducted as a *retrospective* study. Would it not be better if these trials were conducted in a prospective double blind and randomized procedure? The answer is clearly "no". In studying the clearance rate in chronic occlusions, the therapist finds himself in the unique position of not needing the sophisticated statistical tools mandatory for other pharmacologic studies. The reason for this is that the rate of *spontaneous* removals of chronic arterial obstructions can be estimated as nearly zero. Prospective studies, running over years and testing the effect of anticoagulants on the cause of chronic arterial occlusion disease, have not shown one case of spontaneous dissolution of occlusive masses.[17-21,23] Therefore, the study presented here holds that each occlusion removal can be recorded as a real therapeutic success, and that every patient under lytic treatment acts as his own control.

A slightly different view results if we focus on the lytic improvement of narrowings. As evident from recent investigations, the width of chronic arterial narrowings can vary in both directions (constricting and widening) over a period of several weeks or months.[22] However, a definite widening in the course of a 2 day streptokinase treatment (proven by angiography and poststenotic pressure measurements) can likely be, and actually was in this study, regarded as a real therapeutic effect.

Concerning special procedures of streptokinase treatment, no evidence is at hand for the view that SK regimen A (the scheme with which we are most experienced) might be inferior to other regimens (e.g., small dose regimens, minidose regimens, catheter lysis, intermittent regimens, etc.). The schematic way (regimen B: loading dose 250,000 u SK in each case, independent of the individual CAC) is only slightly different from the foregoing one and has the advantage of being more practical than regimens requiring titration of the anti-SK titer prior to treatment. The minor disadvantage of the schematic regimen comprises an insignificant delay in lytic reactions in patients displaying abnormally high CACs (see Chapter 7).

Small dose regimens (30,000 u SK/hr) have been used successfully in the present trial to widen iliac stenoses. Yet, nothing supports the view that small dose procedures are more effective than conventional schemes (100,000 u SK/hr). As shown in Chapter 11, Section III, the period of time for widening stenoses with a low dose regimen was delayed about 1 day compared with high dose regimens. This would match the experience of Gallus et al.[7] and Duckert et al.[28] showing that "the extent of thrombolysis achieved in patients with venous thrombosis was somewhat less than reported by most others using high doses of streptokinase". Furthermore, small dose therapy is far from being free of side effects. Gallus et al.,[7] as well as our group (in a coronary study not yet published), monitored one fatal cerebral bleeding each during this kind of treatment.

Catheter lysis, i.e., the procedure of streptokinase infusion directly into the thrombus material, had been effective in resolving longstanding femoral occlusions (Chapter 11, Section I). One difficult point in this SK-treatment modification was the tendency of thrombus adhesion to the surface of the catheter inserted for 24 hr in the arterial system. Thrombus material, once covering the catheter wall, will inevitably be stripped off upon its removal, thus leading to embolization. In order to avoid such an incident, a strict and uninterrupted anticoagulation procedure (heparin infusion) was necessary. Furthermore, a well-functioning infusion pump counteracting the arterial pressure in the femoral artery must be available.

A retrospective study following up the fates of 67 patients in whom patency of the aorta, the iliac artery and/or the femoral artery was restored by fibrinolytic treatment proved an early reocclusion rate (as seen during hospital stay) of 15%. Later on, the overall rate of reocclusion showed a steady rise reaching 22% at the end of the 3rd year. The incidence then fluctuated around 25% up to the end of the 6th year. Interestingly, there was a striking difference in the fates of iliac and femoral arteries cleared by lytic therapy. After discharge from the hospital, the reocclusion rates of iliac arteries averaged between 0 and 12% over the whole 1 to 6 year observation period, whereas the femoral occlusion figures rose steadily to 50% until the end of the 3rd year. A distinct difference in reocclusion rates was seen between the coagulated and noncoagulated patients in that continuous oral anticoagulants appear to provide effective prophylaxis against reocclusion following lytic occlusion removal.

In conducting streptokinase treatment, side effects have to be taken into account. A compilation of side effects as seen in 600 SK-infusion series was presented. Naturally, cerebral bleeding accidents were of greatest concern to the therapists. A total 0.7% fatal cerebral accidents were recorded, a figure limiting the application of streptokinase treatment to such cases where a clinical success could be expected in a fairly high order of magnitude. The decision as to what rate of clearance expectation should be regarded as a borderline, below which lytic therapy cannot be justified, lies within the responsibility of the attending physician. We estimate a 70%, or higher, probability of vessel clearance as a proper figure for performing streptokinase treatment (e.g., femoral or iliac occlusions up to 2 weeks of age). However, in severe cases where vessel surgery cannot be conducted on the grounds of coronary heart disease, or other severe ailments, a streptokinase treatment might be recommended despite a much lower expectation rate.

REFERENCES

1. Alexander, K., Buhl, U., Holsten, D., Poliwoda, H., and Wagner, H. H., Fibrinolytische Therapie des chronischen Arterienverschlusses, *Med. Klin.*, 63, 2067, 1968.
2. Ehringer, H. and Fischer, M., Erfolgreiche thrombolytische Therapie bei subakuten arteriellen Thrombosen, *Med. Welt*, 1726, 1968.
3. Kaindl, F., Pilgerstorfer, H. W., Weidinger, P., and Fischer, M., Untersuchungen zur Thrombolyse älterer arterieller Verschlüsse mit Streptokinase, *Med. Welt*, 1731, 1968.
4. Schoop, W., Martin, M., and Zeitler, E., Beseitigung von Stenosen in Extremitätenarterien durch intravenöse Streptokinase-Therapie, *Dtsch. Med. Wschr.*, 93, 1629, 1968.
5. Schoop, W., Martin, M., and Zeitler, E., Beseitigung alter Arterienverschlüsse durch intravenöse Streptokinaseinfusion, *Dtsch. Med. Wschr.*, 93, 2312, 1968.
6. Gottlob, R. and Blümel, G., Studies on thrombolysis with streptokinase; I. On the penetration of streptokinase into thrombi, *Thrombos. Diathes. Haemorrh. (Stuttg.)*, 19, 94, 1968.
7. Gottlob, R., Blümel, G., Piza, P., Brücke, P., und Böhmig, H. J., Die Lysierbarkeit operativ gewonnener menschlicher Thromben verschiedenen Alters in Streptokinase, *Wien. Med. Wschr.*, 118, 1, 1968.
8. Gottlob, R., Blümel, G., Piza, P., Brücke, P., and Böhmig, H. J., Studies on thrombolysis with streptokinase; II. The influence of changes due to age in thrombi and whole blood clots, *Thrombos. Diathes. haemorrh. (Stuttg)*, 9, 516, 1968.
9. Jäger, E., Zur pathologischen Anatomie der Thrombangiitis obliterans bei juveniler Extremitätengangrän. 1. und 2. Mitteilung, *Virchows Arch. path. Anat.*, 284, 527, 1932.

10. Klostermeyer, W., Zur Frage der Arterienthrombose unter dem Krankheitsbild der Endangiitis obliterans, *Langenbeck's Arch. klin. Chir.*, 263, 545, 1950.

11. Mittelmeier, H., Pathologische Anatomie der obliterierenden Gefäßerkrankungen, in *Die obliterierenden Gefäßerkrankungen,* Hess, H., Ed., Urban & Schwarzenbach, Berlin, 1959, 1.

12. Rosolleck, H., Lyse von humanen Blutgerinnseln im Reagenzglas, *Klin. Wschr.,* 39, 440, 1961.

13. Rosolleck, H., Zur Wirkungsweise fibrinolytischer Substanzen, *Thrombos. Diathes. Haemorrh. (Stuttg.),* 9, 459, 1963.

14. Le Veen, H. H. and Diaz, C. A., Venous and arterial occlusive disease treated by enzymatic clot lysis, *Arch. Surg.,* 105, 927, 1972.

15. Persson, A. V., Thomson, J. E., and Patman, D., Streptokinase as an adjunct to arterial surgery, *Arch. Surg.,* 107, 779, 1973.

16. Heinrich, F. and Schmutzler, R., Ergebnisse der Thrombolyse-behandlung chronischer Gliedmaßenarterienverschlusse, *Dtsch. Med. J.,* 23, 351, 1972.

17. Tilgren, C., Obliterative arterial disease of the lower limbs. IV. Evaluation of long-term anticoagulant therapy, *Acta Med. Scand.,* 178, 203, 1965.

18. Tilgren, C., Stenson, S., and Lund, F., Obliterative arterial disease of the lower limbs studied by means of repeated femoral arteriography, *Acta Radial. (Stockholm),* 1, 1161, 1963.

19. Hess, H., Anticoagulant therapy of peripheral arterial thrombosis, in *Pathogenesis and Treatment of Thromboembolic Diseases,* Koller, F., Duckert, F., and Streuli, F.,, Eds., F. K. Schattauer-Verlag, Stuttgart, 1966, 371.

20. Richards, R. R. and Begg, T. B., Long-term anticoagulant therapy in atherosclerotic peripheral disease, *Vasc. Dis. (N.Y.),* 4, 27, 1967.

21. Burghalter, A., Widmer, L. K., and Glaus, L., Chronischer Gliedmaßenarterienverschulß und Langzeitantikoagulation, *Vasa,* 3, 185, 1974.

22. Schoop, W. and Schmidtke, I., Spontane Lumenerweiterungen von Arterienstenosen, *Herz/Kreisl.,* 5, 9, 1973.

23. Lund, F. and Tilgren, C., Anticoagulant therapy in occlusive peripheral arterial disease and its evaluation, in *Pathogenesis and Treatment of Thromboembolic Disease,* Koller, F., Duckert, F. and Streuli, F., Eds., F. K. Schattauer-Verlag, Stuttgart, 1966, 385.

24. Deutsch, E. and Ehringer, H., Thrombolytic therapy in chronic arterial occlusions, *J. Clin. Pathol.,* 25, 644, 1972.

25. Verstraete, M., Vermylen, J., and Donati, M. B., The effect of streptokinase on chronic arterial occlusions and stenoses, *Ann. Int. Med.,* 74, 377, 1971.

26. Martin, M., Schoop, W., and Zeitler, E., *Thrombolyse bei chronischer Arteriopathie,* Verlag Hans Huber, Bern, 1970.

27. Gallus, A. S., Hirsch, J., Cade, J. F., Turpie, A. G. G., Walker, I. R., and Gent, M., Thrombolysis with a combination of small doses of streptokinase and full doses of heparin, *Semin. Thrombos. Hemost.,* 2, 14, 1975.

28. Duckert, F., Marbet, G. A., Walter, M., Six, P., Nyman, D., Madar, G., da Silva, M. A., Widmer, L. K., Schmitt, H. E., and Vokal, J., Thrombolytic treatment with a streptokinase low dose regimen, in *New Concepts in Streptokinase Dosimetry,* Martin, M., Schoop, W., and Hirsch, J., Eds., Hans Huber, Bern, 1978.

Chapter 16

LABORATORY PROCEDURES FOR MONITORING STREPTOKINASE TREATMENT

I. EQUIPMENT

Coagulometer — according to Schnitger and Gross,[2] manufactured by H. Amelung KG, Lemgo-Brake, West Germany. The coagulometer is used for determining coagulation times in a variety of tests. In principle, blood samples are "crocheted" automatically by two parallel wire hooks. A current circuit is closed when the first fibrin thread appears, which stops the crocheting mechanism. Digital read-off of the coagulation time.

Thromboelastograph — according to Hartert,[1] manufactured by Hellige AG, Freiburg/Br., West Germany. The mechanism of the thromboelastograph is as follows (Figure 1): a cylindrical piston suspended from the torsion wire dips into a small steel cuvette containing the specimen for coagulation and/or lysis. A moving device rotates the cuvette over an angle of 4°45′, at the same time swinging it to and fro. Each torsion phase of the cuvette lasts 9 sec, including a rest period of 1 sec in each end position. The suspended piston dipping into the rotating curvette filled with clottable material starts to turn in the same rhythm due to the formation of elastic fibrin fibers during the clotting process. The rotations become increasingly stronger the more solid the clot gets. A mirror attached to the torsion wire is also rotated proportionately. The light ray reflected from the mirror falls onto a millimeter scale and, via an image lens, onto a light-sensitive chart traveling past the lens at a speed of 2 mm/min. The intensity of the reflected light ray and the light sensitivity of the chart are so adjusted that the chart is sufficiently exposed only at the turning points of the rotation as the light ray pauses for a second. Before clotting of the specimen occurs, there is a straight line. When the clotting process starts, this straight line divides into two symmetrical branches. Thus an envelope curve — the thromboelastogram — appears on the chart. After clot lysis has succeeded, the branches recede again to a straight line. The sequence of straight line (sample is unclotted), deviation of the branches (clotting), and renewed approach to a straight line (lysis) gives the TEG curve a spindle-shaped configuration.

- **Water bath** — 37°C and 56°C.
- **Incubator** — 37°C.
- **Drier** — 85°C.
- **Nissl tubes** — "Resistance", manufactured by Rudolf Maurer, Lorsbach/ Taunus, West Germany.
- **Microliter -Marburg - Pipettes** — manufactured by Eppendorg Gerätebau, Netheler & Hinz, Hamburg, West Germany.
- **Filter paper** — Rundfilter No. 595, diameter 11 cm, manufactured by Schleicher & Schüll, Einbeck, West Germany.
- **Double logarithmic paper** — No. 369-1/2:1, manufactured by Schleicher & Schüll, Einbeck, West Germany.

II. GENERAL PROCEDURES

A. Plasma Preparation

Mix 9 mℓ native blood with 1 mℓ of 3.8% sodium citrate solution. Spin at 2500 r/ min. Pipette off the plasma.

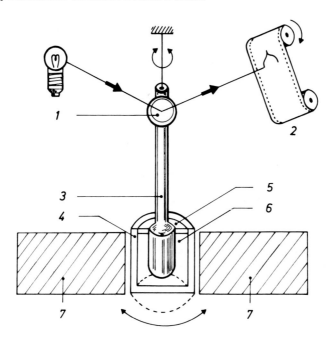

FIGURE 1.   Thromboelastograph, according to Hartert[1]. 1 = mirror attached to shaft of piston and torsion wire; 2 = light sensitive chart; 3 = piston shaft connected with torsion wire; 4 = steel cuvette; 5 = paraffin layer; 6 = specimen coagulating and lysing in the cuvette; 7 = heated metal bar For further details, see text.

B. Euglobulin Preparation: Modification of the Method According to Von Kaulla and McDonald[4]

The citrated blood of 20 healthy volunteers was mixed and stored at −20°C. On the day when an experiment was scheduled, 6 tubes each with 1.5 mℓ of the thawed, pooled plasma were prepared. After adding 22.5 mℓ distilled water, each mixture was exposed to carbon dioxide vapor for 6 min. Thereafter, the solution was centrifuged for 10 min at 2500 r/min, the supernatant decanted, and the euglobulin precipitate dissolved in 0.27 mℓ Michaelis buffer pH 7.8 and 0.03 mℓ 5% EDTA solution. The resultant mixture containing euglobulin from 1.5 mℓ plasma dissolved in 0.3 mℓ EDTA buffer equaled a 500% euglobulin solution. The corresponding EDTA concentration was 0.013 mol/ℓ.

C. Preparation of a Mixed Bovine Fibrinogen-Plasminogen Solution

The content of one flask of bovine fibrinogen (60 mg) was dissolved in 6 mℓ Michaelis buffer pH 7.8. In order to bring this about, the fibrinogen powder was transferred into a glass tube and topped with 5.0 mℓ Michaelis buffer. Complete dissolution was regularly recorded after 30 min incubation in a water bath at 37°C. The fibrinogen solution was then filtered, using folding filter, Type 595-1/2, leading to a 1000 mg% bovine fibrinogen solution. In a previous study,[3] it was shown that Behringwerke bovine fibrinogen preparation was rich in bovine plasminogen. The ratio of plasminogen to fibrinogen was, on the average, 2.7 times higher than in human plasma.

D. Preparation of a 16 u/mℓ Thrombin Solution

The contents of one "Antithrombin Reagenz" ampoule (Hoffmann-LaRoche AG, Grenzach/Baden, West Germany), i.e., 16 u thrombin, was dissolved in 1 mℓ Michaelis buffer pH 7.4.

E. Preparation of a 1000, 2000, or 8000 u/ml Streptokinase Solution

Dissolve 5000 u of streptokinase (1 flask of test streptokinase, Behringwerke AG, Marburg/Lahn, West Germany) in either 5 ml, 2.5 ml or 0.65 ml of Michaelis buffer pH 7.4, yielding a 1000, 2000, or 8000 u SK/ml solution.

F. Preparation of a 5% EDTA Solution

Dissolve 5 g of the disodium salt of ethylenediaminetetraacetic acid (EDTA) in 100 ml of distilled water. This results in a 5%, or 0.134 mol/l, or 0.268 val/l EDTA solution.

III. DETERMINATION OF CAC (CIRCULATING ANTI-SK CONTENT) (DEUTSCH AND FISCHER[5])

A. Principle of Test

Each individual suffers streptococci infections and, therefore, produces antibodies against a wide spectrum of streptococci antigens. The antigen of interest in connection with SK therapy is antistreptokinase. Antistreptokinase inhibits streptokinase at an approximately linear ratio, i.e., 100,000 anti-SK units "neutralize" 100,000 u SK, and 1 million anti-SK u about 1 million u SK. However, this rule applies *cum grano salis*. During infusion of a loading dose equaling the exact amount of CAC as determined by the Deutsch and Fischer test, some lytic reactions were already seen prior to the influx of the whole neutralizing dose. Yet, major effects, such as full plasminogen depletion or a definite rise in measurable streptokinase and activator quantities, were not recorded before administration of the full CAC equivalent (see Chapter 7, Sections VIII and IX). Therefore, anti-SK titer titration and administration of the corresponding SK amount as loading dose seem, to us, a prerequisite for properly conducting streptokinase treatment.

B. Steps in Performance of Method

Dissolution of 5000 u streptokinase in 2.5 ml of 0.9% NaCl solution (= stock solution). Six tubes are arrayed and coded No. 1 through 6. One ml of saline solution is pipetted into each of tubes 2 through 6. One ml of the stock solution (containing 2000 u SK/ml) is transferred into tubes 1 and 2. One ml of the mixture of tube 2 is pipetted into tube 3. One ml of the mixture of tube 3 is pipetted into tube 4, and so forth. The final concentration in each tube is as follows:

- No.1. 2000 u SK/ml
- No.2. 1000 u SK/ml
- No.3. 500 u SK/ml
- No.4. 250 u SK/ml
- No.5. 125 u SK/ml
- No.6. 62.5 u SK/ml

Another six test tubes are arrayed and coded A through F, then 0.1 ml streptokinase solution is transferred from tube 1 to tube A, 0.1 ml from tube 2 to tube B, 0.1 ml from tube 3 to tube C, and so on.

Subsequently, 1 ml of citrated blood (1 + 9) was pipetted into each of tubes A to F. This resulted in streptokinase concentrations of:

- 200 u/ml blood in tube A
- 100 u/ml blood in tube B
- 50 u/ml blood in tube C

- 25   u/ml blood in tube D
- 12.5   u/ml blood in tube E
- 6.25 u/ml blood in tube F

Then 0.1 ml of a thrombin solution (10 u/ml) is pipetted into tubes A to F. After coagulation, the clots are incubated 10 min at 37°C. After this time, evaluation is made of the streptokinase concentration in the tube where lysis occurred next to one in which no clot dissolution was registered. The respective streptokinase concentration/ml blood is multiplied by the blood volume (kg weight × 70). The resulting streptokinase value, supposed to represent the antistreptokinase content, is called "circulating anti-SK content" (CAC).

IV. ACTIVATOR DETERMINATION (MARTIN[6])

A. Principle of Test (Figure 2)

Chemically, activator is defined as the stoichiometric complex of human plasminogen and streptokinase. Activator is thought to be the decisive compound in activating bovine, and probably also human plasminogen, thus mediating thrombus dissolution.

Activator measurement is based on clot lysis time as recorded by the thromboelastograph. The test clot constituents are bovine fibrinogen, bovine plasminogen (present in the bovine fibrinogen preparation), EDTA, and human plasma containing activator (SK-plg-complex), the concentration of which is to be measured in this test.

The principle of measurement is based on the fact that bovine plasminogen adsorbed on bovine fibrin can be converted into proteolytic bovine plasmin by either the equimolar streptokinase-human plasminogen complex (activator) or urokinase. This means that the quantity of plasmin produced, and thus the lysis time of a bovine fibrin test clot formed in the presence of activator or urokinase, is directly dependent on the quantity of activator or urokinase employed. Therefore, the test clot lysis time is inversely related to the activator or urokinase concentrations.

B. Steps in Performance of Method (Figures 3 and 4)

1. "Adjustment" of Fibrinogen Solution

For measurement of clot lysis times, the thromboelastographic technique of Hartert[1] was applied.

A 1 ml tuberculin syringe was filled with the following mixture:

- 0.10 ml bovine fibrinogen solution 1000 mg%
- 0.05 ml EDTA solution 0.5%
- 0.05 ml NaCl solution 0.9%
- 0.05 ml thrombin solution (16 u/ml)

The mixture was quickly transferred into a preheated TEG cuvette and the TEG piston turned down. A paraffin cover was applied. The resultant spindle width (as monitored on the observation millimeter scale) had to be between 0.3 and 0.5 cm. Where the spindle width exceeded 0.5 cm, the fibrinogen solution had to be "adjusted", i.e., diluted further, and monitored until this range was reached.

In earlier investigations,[8] a linear relation was found between spindle width and fibrin content of the clot. Adjustment of the spindle width (by changing the fibrin content of the clot) is therefore consistent with adjustment of the fibrin concentration of the clot.

The syringe was cleaned after each measurement by the following procedure. Distilled water was drawn up in and blown out of the syringe five times. Thereafter, 0.1

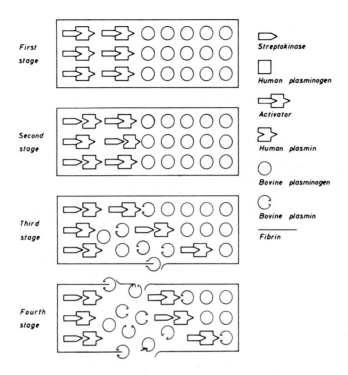

First stage

Second stage

Third stage

Fourth stage

Streptokinase

Human plasminogen

Activator

Human plasmin

Bovine plasminogen

Bovine plasmin

Fibrin

FIGURE 2. Basic interactions constituting the activator determination assay. When activator enters the system of bovine fibrin and plasminogen in the test clot, lysis of the clot starts at once. The clot lysis time is inversely correlated with the amount of activator added. Note that part of the activator is dissociated into its inert (with respect to plasminogen-plasmin conversion) plasmin and streptokinase compounds.

mℓ of the fibrinogen solution was drawn up and likewise discarded. The syringe was then filled in the way depicted above.

2. Plotting of the Standardization Curve

Three samples containing different urokinase concentrations were needed (Urokinase, Leo Pharmaceutical Products Ltd., Ballerup, Denmark). The 3160 CTA-u urokinase was dissolved in 1.05 mℓ saline solution to obtain a 3000 u/mℓ solution. Then 0.1 mℓ of the latter was diluted with 0.9 mℓ saline solution to obtain a 300 u/mℓ solution, 0.1 mℓ of this mixture was diluted with 0.9 mℓ saline solution to obtain a 30 u/mℓ solution, and 0.1 mℓ of the latter was further diluted with 0.9 mℓ saline solution leading to a 3 u/mℓ solution.

The following mixture was drawn up into a 1 mℓ tuberculin syringe:

- 0.10 mℓ "adjusted" bovine fibrinogen solution
- 0.05 mℓ EDTA solution
- 0.05 mℓ urokinase solution containing 3 CTA-u, 30 CTA-u, and 300 CTA-u/mℓ
- 0.05 mℓ thrombin solution

The mixture was immediately injected into a TEG steel cuvette and the lysis time recorded. In order to arrive at the clot lysis times, the spindle-shaped TEG lysis curves were measured by determining the distance between the point where the spindle begins to widen beyond 1 mm and the point where it recedes to 1 mm. The values thus ob-

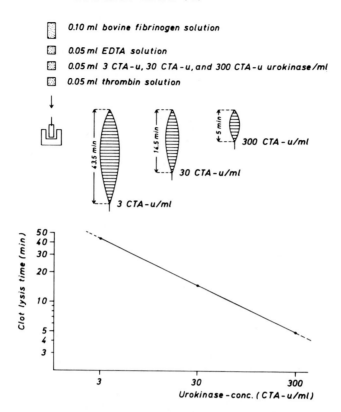

FIGURE 3.   Schematic representation of quantitative activator determination in the plasma of patients. I. Drawing the standardization line. For reference, defined amounts of urokinase were dissolved in saline solution.

tained, divided by 2, gave the test clot lysis time in minutes. The respective lysis times were entered on the ordinate and the related urokinase concentrations plotted on the abscissa of double logarithmic paper. The respective points were connected by a straight line representing the standardization line.

3. Determination of Activator Expressed in Terms of Urokinase Equivalents (CTA-u/ m*ℓ*)

The following mixture was drawn up into a tuberculin syringe:

- 0.10 m*ℓ* "adjusted bovine fibrinogen solution
- 0.05 m*ℓ* EDTA solution
- 0.05 m*ℓ* undiluted plasma of patients undergoing treatment with streptokinase infusion
- 0.05 m*ℓ* thrombin solution

The mixture was quickly transferred into a preheated TEG cuvette. Coagulation and clot dissolution were recorded. The clot lysis time was read off the TEG chart. The lysis time, in minutes, was located on the standardization line and read in "CTA-u/ m*ℓ*".

Methodic variation: 100 ± 20 CTA-u/m*ℓ*

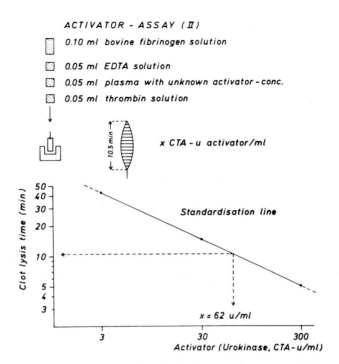

FIGURE 4. Schematic representation of quantitative activator determination in the plasma of patients. II. Measurement of activator concentration in the patient plasma under streptokinase therapy in terms of urokinase equivalent.

V. PLASMINOGEN DETERMINATION[7,9]

A. Principle of Test (Figure 5)

The method employed is based upon the conversion of plasminogen into activator by large and constant amounts of streptokinase. Activator contained in a standard coagulum consisting of bovine fibrinogen, bovine plasminogen, streptokinase, and a 1:40 dilution of human plasma converts bovine plasminogen into plasmin. Lysis of test coagulum is hereby induced. The speed of lysis is limited by the concentration of activator incorporated in the test coagulum. The variable component of the activator being human plasminogen, the speed of lysis is directly dependent upon the concentration of human plasminogen present in the standard coagulum.

Both plasminogen and plasmin, its activated form, are exchangeable in the test, i.e., plasminogen determination performed by the activator assay is unable to differentiate between plasminogen and plasmin. Neither anti-SK titers up to a circulating antibody content of 2 million, nor antiplasmin activities in the patient's plasma, interfere with this test.

B. Steps in Performance of Method (Figures 6 and 7)

1. "Adjustment" of Fibrinogen Solution

For measurement of clot lysis times the thromboelastographic technique of Hartert[1] was applied.

A 1 mℓ tuberculin syringe was filled with the following mixture:

- 0.10 mℓ bovine fibrinogen solution 1000 mg%
- 0.05 mℓ Michaelis buffer pH 7.4
- 0.05 mℓ streptokinase solution (8000 u/mℓ)
- 0.05 mℓ thrombin solution (16 u/mℓ)

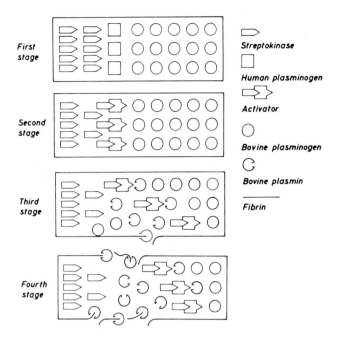

FIGURE 5.   Schematic representation of plasminogen determination procedure by adopting the activator method. In the test clot, human plasminogen molecules meet streptokinase molecules, thus forming activator (equimolar = SK-human plasminogen complex). The latter converts bovine plasminogen to plasmin, leading to clot dissolution. The higher human plasminogen concentration is present in the clot, the quicker lysis takes place.

This mixture was blown out from the tuberculin syringe into the TEG steel cuvette which had been preheated on the thromboelastograph. The TEG piston was let down, a paraffin cover applied, and the spindle-shaped TEG curve of coagulation and lysis recorded. The resulting spindle width was to be between 0.7 and 1.0 cm. Where this width was found to have been exceeded, the fibrinogen solution had to be "adjusted", i.e., diluted further, and monitored in the TEG until this value was reached.

In earlier investigations,[8] a linear relation was found between spindle width and fibrin content of the clot. Adjustment of the spindle width (by changing the fibrin content of the clot) is therefore consistent with adjustment of the fibrin concentration of the clot.

The syringe was cleaned after each measurement by the following procedure. Distilled water was drawn up in and blown out of the syringe five times. Thereafter, 0.1 mℓ of the fibrinogen solution was drawn up and likewise discarded. The syringe was then filled in the way depicted above.

2. Determination of Test Clot Lysis Times with Known Plasminogen Concentrations (Standardization)

Pooled plasma of 60 healthy volunteers was diluted 1:40, 1:200, 1:1000, 1:5000, 1:25,000 and 1:125,000. The 1:40 dilution was called "100% plasminogen solution", the 1:200 dilution 20%, the 1:1000 dilution 4%, the 1:5000 dilution 0.8%, the 1:25,000 dilution 0.16% and the 1:125,000 dilution referred to as "0.03% plasminogen solution".

A standard clot was produced by drawing the following mixture into a tuberculin syringe:

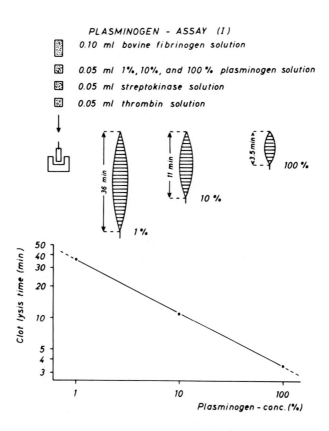

FIGURE 6.   Schematic representation of plasminogen measurement.
I. Steps for constructing the calibration line.

- 0.10 ml "adjusted" fibrinogen solution
- 0.05 ml 100%, 20%, 4%, 0.8%, 0.16% or 0.03% plasminogen solution
- 0.05 ml streptokinase solution (8000 u/ml)
- 0.05 ml thrombin solution (16 u/ml)

The mixtures were immediately injected into the TEG cuvette and the lysis time was registered. In order to evaluate the clot lysis times, the spindle-shape thromboelasto-graph lysis curves were measured by determining the distance between the point where the spindle begins to widen out from 1 mm onwards, and the point where it recedes to 1 mm. The values thus obtained, divided by 2, gave the test clot lysis times in minutes. The resulting six lysis times were entered on the ordinate and the related plasminogen concentrations plotted on the abscissa of double logarithmic paper. The resulting points were connected by a straight line to obtain a standard line.

As all standard values ranging from 100% down to 0.03% plasminogen were located on a straight line on the double logarithmic system, only two standard values (of 100% and 1%) were needed for routine determinations.

3. Determination of Unknown Plasma Plasminogen Concentration
The following mixture was drawn into a tuberculin syringe:

- 0.10 ml "adjusted" bovine fibrinogen solution
- 0.05 ml 1:40 diluted human plasma
- 0.05 ml streptokinase solution (8000 u/ml)
- 0.05 ml thrombin solution (16 u/ml)

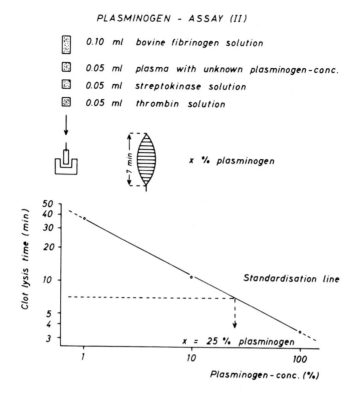

FIGURE 7.   Schematic representation of plasminogen measurement.
II. Steps for determining unknown plasminogen concentrations.

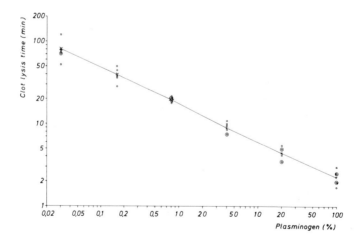

FIGURE 8.   Standardization line obtained from clot lysis times of six
different normal plasma samples.

The lysis time was registered on the thromboelastograph and the plasminogen concentration read on the standard line in percent of normal.

Methodic variations: $100 \pm 13.2\%$,
$$1 \pm 0.35\%,$$
$$0.01 \pm 0.0068\%.$$

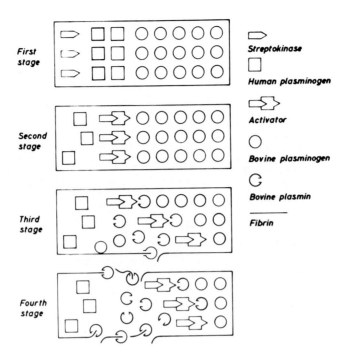

FIGURE 9. Schematic representation of the sequence of events during performance of the streptokinase determination assay. Small amounts of streptokinase are added to a fixed excess of human plasminogen, bovine plasminogen, and bovine fibrin in the standard clot. Streptokinase quickly combines with human plasminogen to form activator. Activator itself converts bovine plasminogen to plasmin, the latter of which digests the fibrin component of the clot. There is an inverse relationship between streptokinase concentration and lysis time of the clot. Thus different lysis times indicate various streptokinase concentrations.

VI. QUANTITATIVE STREPTOKINASE MEASUREMENT IN PLASMA OF PATIENTS UNDERGOING FIBRINOLYTIC TREATMENT[8,11]

A. Principle of Test (Figure 9)

The principle of this method is based on the clot lysis time as recorded by the thromboelastograph. The test clot constituents are bovine fibrin, bovine plasminogen, human euglobulin, EDTA, human plasma (with unknown streptokinase quantity) and thrombin. As human plasminogen (euglobulin) and fibrinogen are present in the test coagulum in rather high concentrations (fixed excess), no interference with changing plasminogen and fibrinogen levels of the patient plasma was observed. Further, due to high EDTA concentrations, no interaction with platelet functions and coagulation factors took place.

B. Steps in Performance of Method (Figures 10 and 11)

1. "Adjustment" of a Bovine Fibrinogen Solution

The streptokinase determination performed here was carried out by a clot lysis time method registered in the thromboelastograph according to Hartert.[1] In order to obtain equivalent clot lysis time, standardized tracings with a constant width of the spindle-shaped envelope curves were necessary.

The adjustment procedure was as follows: Draw up in a tuberculin syringe:

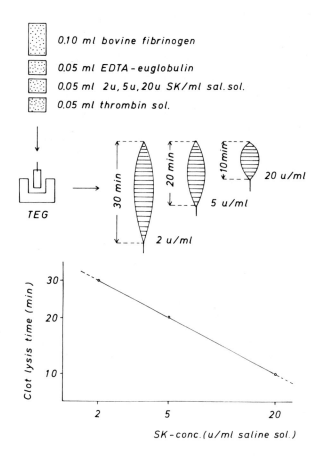

FIGURE 10.   Schematic representation of quantitative SK determination method. I. Drawing of standardization line.

- 0.10 mℓ bovine fibrinogen solution 1000 mg%
- 0.05 mℓ EDTA-euglobulin solution 500%
- 0.05 mℓ Michaelis buffer pH 7.4
- 0.05 mℓ thrombin solution (16 u/mℓ)

The mixture was quickly transferred into a preheated TEG cuvette and the TEG piston turned down. A paraffin cover was applied. The resulting spindle width was to have been between 0.3 and 0.5 cm. Where this width was exceeded, the fibrinogen solution had to be "adjusted", i.e., diluted further and monitored in the TEG until this value range was reached.

2. Standardization Line

Four samples containing different streptokinase concentrations were needed. A 5000 u quantity of streptokinase was dissolved in 5 mℓ of a 0.9% sodium chloride solution, resulting in a 1000 u/mℓ streptokinase solution. From this streptokinase stock solution, concentrations of 2 u, 5 u, and 20 u were prepared using a 0.9% sodium chloride solution as solvent.

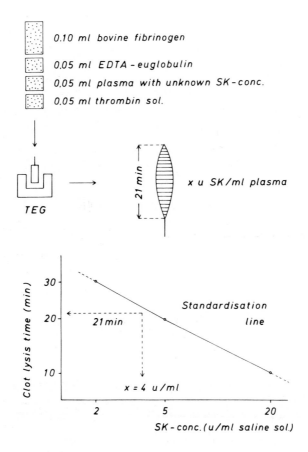

FIGURE 11.   Schematic representation of quantitative SK determination method. II. Measurement of SK concentration in the patient plasma.

The following mixture was drawn into a 1 m*l* tuberculin syringe:

- 0.10 m*l* "adjusted" bovine fibrinogen solution
- 0.05 m*l* EDTA-euglobulin solution 500%
- 0.05 m*l* streptokinase solution containing 2 u, 5 u, or 20 u streptokinase/m*l*, respectively
- 0.05 m*l* thrombin solution (16 u/m*l*)

The mixture was immediately injected into a TEG steel cuvette and the lysis times registered. In order to determine the clot lysis times, the spindle-shaped TEG lysing curves were measured by determining the distance between the point where the spindle begins to widen from 1 mm onwards and the point where it recedes to 1 mm. The values thus obtained, divided by 2, gave the test clot lysis times in minutes. The lysis times were entered on the ordinate and the related streptokinase concentrations on the abscissa of double logarithmic paper. The respective points were connected by a straight line, resulting in the standardization line (Figures 11 and 12).

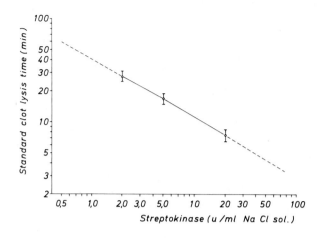

FIGURE 12.   Standardization line derived from values of ten SK assays. Brackets indicate standard deviations.

3. Determination of an Unknown Streptokinase Concentration in the Plasma
The following mixture was drawn into a tuberculin syringe:

- 0.10 mℓ "adjusted" bovine fibrinogen solution
- 0.05 mℓ EDTA-euglobulin solution
- 0.05 mℓ patient plasma (undiluted)
- 0.05 mℓ thrombin solution

The lysis time was recorded in the thromboelastograph and the streptokinase concentration read on the standardization line.

Methodic variations: 2 ± 0.19 u SK/mℓ,
5 ± 0.47 u SK/mℓ,
20 ± 2.5 u SK/mℓ.

VII. PLASMIN ASSAY[8,10]

A. Principle of Test
Plasmin-containing plasma, 0.05 mℓ, was pipetted onto a plasminogen-free bovine fibrin film. Upon incubation at 37°C, smaller or larger lysis areas were produced, depending upon the sample's plasmin concentration. The lysis area value calculated by planimetric methods was a relative index of plasmin activity. Quantification was possible by applying a calibration line. For this purpose, defined porcine plasminogen standardized in novo-u/mℓ, produced by NOVO Industri A/S, Copenhagen, Denmark) were tested on the fibrin plates parallel to the plasmin aliquots. The resulting lysis area values were entered on the ordinate and the respective novo-u/mℓ figures on the abscissa of a double logarithmic paper. The resulting points were connected and gave the calibration line. Thereafter, each lysis area value could easily be transformed into novo-u/mℓ.

B. Steps in Performance of Method

1.   Plasminogen-free bovine fibrin plates, according to Lassen,[10] were produced as follows: 120 mg bovine fibrinogen (Behringwerke AG, Marburg/Lahn, West Germany) were transferred into a test tube and topped by 10 mℓ veronal buffer

pH 7.8, then incubated at 37°C for 1 hr. Transfer into an Erlenmeyer flask and add veronal buffer up to 40 mℓ. Filtration of the fibrinogen solution then performed with filter 595, diameter 11 cm (Schleicher & Schüll, Dassel, Kreis Einbeck, West Germany). Then 3000 u thrombin (Topostasin®, Hoffmann-La Roche AG, Grenzach/Baden, West Germany) was dissolved in 6 mℓ physiological saline solution; 0.5 mℓ of this solution was further diluted 1:10 (0.5 mℓ + 4.5 mℓ), resulting in a 50 u thrombin/mℓ solution.

Seven Erlenmeyer flasks of 25 mℓ volume, coded I to VII, and seven Petri dishes (10 cm diameter), coded A to G, were arrayed. A 0.4 mℓ quantity of thrombin solution was pipetted into Flask I to VII each. Under rotating movements of Flask I, 8 mℓ fibrinogen solution was added. Immediately transfer the thrombin-fibrinogen solution into Petri Dish A. The same was done with Flask II and Dish B, Flask III and Dish C, etc. The Petri dishes were closed by a lid, in the inner side of which a filter paper had been fixed. The dishes were incubated at 37°C for 1 hr, after which period a solid fibrin film had developed. The last step consisted of heating the plate at 85°C for 45 min. The fibrin plates remained stable in the refrigerator at +4°C up to 1 week. To prove that the fibrin film was free from plasminogen, 0.05 mℓ of a 100 u/mℓ urokinase solution (Leo Pharmaceutical Products Ltd., Ballerup, Denmark) were pipetted onto the fibrin film. It was mandatory that no lysis occurred after incubation at 37°C for 18 hr.

2. The *plasmin assay* was conducted as follows: 1 mℓ of an 0.9% NaCl solution was pipetted into a test tube containing 2 novo-u of porcine plasmin. This stock solution of 2 novo-u/mℓ was further diluted 1:8, 1:16, 1:32, and 1:64. Then 0.05 mℓ of plasmin solutions with the respective concentrations of 0.25 u/mℓ, 0.12 u/mℓ and 0.03 u/mℓ were pipetted onto the fibrin plate. Additionally, 0.05 mℓ of plasma with unknown plasmin activity was placed on the plate. After 18 hr incubation at 37°C, or 1 hr at 40°C, the lysis areas were measured planimetrically. The lysis area values were entered on the ordinate and the respective plasmin concentrations on the abscissa of double logarithmic paper to obtain a standardization line. By using the latter, the lysis area produced by a plasma with unknown plasmin concentration was easily converted into "novo-units plasmin/ mℓ".

VIII. FIBRINOGEN DETERMINATION: GRAVIMETRIC METHOD[12]

A. Principle of Test

Citrated plasma was coagulated by adding CaCl$_2$. The resultant fibrin clot was washed, dried, and weighed. The clot weight corresponded to the fibrinogen content of the plasma prior to coagulation.

B. Steps in Performance of Method

Citrated plasma, 2 mℓ, plus 0.2 mℓ of Trasylol® (an antiplasmin to stop further fibrinogenolytic reaction), plus 2 mℓ of CaCl$_2$ solution (0.025 *M*) were mixed and incubated at 37°C for 2 hr. Subsequently, the resultant clot was washed in physiologic saline solution and distilled water. It was then dried on filter paper, bathed twice each in 96% alcohol and in ether, and dried again in the incubator at 37°C overnight, following which the dried clot was weighed on an analytical scale. The quantity measured was multiplied by 100 and divided by 1.8, resulting in mg% plasma fibrinogen.

Standard values: 409 ± 71 mg%.

IX. FIBRINOGEN DETERMINATION: HEAT PRECIPITATION METHOD[13]

A. Principle of Test

Fibrinogen is a heat-labile protein and is precipitated by heating citrated plasma at 56°C.

B. Steps in Performance of Method

Citrated plasma, 1.0 mℓ, is pipetted into a calibrated Nissl tube and incubated for 10 min at 56°C. The precipitate settles at 2000 r/min. According to a table provided by Schulz,[13] the volume of the sediment corresponds to the amount of plasma fibrinogen in mg%.

Standard values: 357 mg% ± 55 mg%.

X. DETERMINATION OF FIBRINOGEN CONCENTRATION: THROMBIN TIME METHOD[14]

A. Principle of Test

Thrombin mediates fibrinogen-fibrin conversion. In a sample containing a fixed and relatively high concentration of thrombin and a varying and relatively small concentration of fibrinogen, the resultant coagulation time will be entirely controlled by the level of fibrinogen present in the system.

B. Steps in Performance of Method

All determinations were carried out with the fibrinogen determination set of Merz & Dade, Munich, West Germany: 0.1 mℓ of citrated plasma (1:10) + 0.9 mℓ of veronal buffer pH 7.35 gave a 1:10 plasma dilution; 0.2 mℓ of this solution was preheated for 2 min at 37°C and clotted by adding 0.1 mℓ of thrombin solution (100 u/mℓ). The clotting time was read off a standard curve in mg% fibrinogen. When the clotting time exceeded 50 sec (corresponding to a fibrinogen value of less than 40 mg%), the determination was repeated with a plasma dilution of 1:5. In this case, the fibrinogen value obtained by means of the standard curve had to be divided by 2. When the clotting time was still longer than 50 sec (corresponding to a fibrinogen value of less than 20 mg%), the plasma was diluted 1:2 and the resultant fibrinogen value had to be divided by 5.

The standard curve was obtained as follows. Dilute a fibrinogen standard solution with veronal buffer to 1:5, 1:15 and 1:40. The determination scheme depicted above was then used for obtaining reference coagulation times. The latter were entered on the ordinate and the respective fibrinogen concentrations in mg% on the abscissa of a double logarithmic paper. This led to a calibration line suited for the reading of plasma-fibrinogen concentrations.

Standard values: 396 ± 73 mg%.

XI. DETERMINATION OF PARTIAL THROMBOPLASTIN TIME (PTT)[15]

A. Principle of Test

PTT measures the intrinsic way of coagulation by kaolin activation of the Hageman factor and addition of platelet factor 3. PTT is abnormally lengthened by coagulation inhibitors, such as heparin or fibrinogen degradation products, and by endogenous clotting defects such as pathological decreases in factors I, II, V, VIII, IX, X, XI and XII.

B. Steps in Performance of Method

A 0.2 mℓ quantity of citrated plasma is incubated with 0.2 mℓ PTT reagent (Behringwerke AG, Marburg/Lahn, West Germany) for 120 sec at 37°C. Subsequently, it is recalcified with 0.2 mℓ of a 0.025 M calcium chloride solution and onset of coagulation determined.

Standard values: 41 ± 3.8 sec.

XII. DETERMINATION OF WHOLE BLOOD RECALCIFICATION TIME

A. Principle of Test

Whole blood recalcification time determines the overall clotting ability encompassing most of the procoagulant factors involved. Furthermore the test responds to inhibition of fibrinogen-fibrin conversion due to the presence of heparin and/or fibrinogen degradation products.

B. Steps in Performance

0.5 mℓ citrated patient blood is given into a glass test tube which is placed into a water bath at 37°C. Subsequently 0.5 mℓ 0.025 M calcium chloride solution is added. The coagulation time is determined.

Standard values: 102 ± 11 sec.

XIII. DETERMINATION OF REPTILASE TIME (RT)[17]

A. Principle of Test

Reptilase (Boehringer, Mannheim, West Germany) is a snake venom enzyme of Bothrops atrox. The venom exerts thrombin-like properties and coagulates plasma by direct fibrinogen-fibrin conversion. This reaction is not influenced by heparin but delayed by fibrinogen degradation products (FDP). Further, fibrinogen depression leads to lengthening of RT.

B. Steps in Performance

A 0.3 mℓ quantity of plasma was incubated at 37°C for 120 sec and 0.1 mℓ of Reptilase reagent (contents of 1 flask dissolved in 1 mℓ distilled water) added. Clotting time was then determined.

Standard values: 13 ± 1.9 sec.

XIV. DETERMINATION OF REPTILASE TIME CORRECTED FOR FIBRINOGEN (cRT)

A. Principle of Test

As outlined in Section XIII, the reptilase time is dependent on both the fibrinogen concentration and circulating fibrinogen degradation products (FDP). In order to measure the influence of FDP exclusively, plasma of a normal fibrinogen level was added to the assay.

B. Steps in Performance

A 0.15 mℓ quantity of normal plasma and 0.15 mℓ of patient plasma are incubated for 120 sec at 37°C. After that, 0.1 mℓ reptilase reagent is added and the coagulation time determined.

Standard values: 13 ± 1.9 sec.

REFERENCES

1. **Hartert, H.,** Die Thromboelastographie. Eine Methode zur physikalischen Analyse des Blutgerinnungs vorgangs, *Z. Ges. Exp. Med.,* 117, 189, 1951.
2. **Schnitger, H. and Gross, R.,** Über ein Universalgerät zur automatischen Registrierung von Gerinnungs zeiten, *Klin. Wochenschr.,* 32, 1011, 1954.
3. **Auel, H. and Martin, M.,** Plasminogengehalt eines im Handel befindlichen Rinderfibrinogens, *Z. Klin. Chemie Klin. Biochem.,* 12, 385, 1974.
4. **Von Kaulla, K. N. and McDonald, T. S.,** The effect of heparin on components of the human fibrinolytic system, *Blood,* 13, 811, 1958.
5. **Deutsch, E. and Fischer, M.,** Die Wirkung intravenös applizierter Streptokinase auf Fibrinolyse und Blutgerinnung, *Thrombos. Diathes. Haemorrh. (Stuttg.),* 6, 482, 1960.
6. **Martin, M.,** Investigation of activator kinetics in undiluted plasma in terms of Urokinase equivalents, *Thrombos. Diathes. Haemorrh. (Stuttg.),* 36, 566, 1976.
7. **Martin, M.,** Semiquantitative Plasminogenbestimmung mit Hilfe des Thrombelastographen. Eine Methode zur Kontrolle der Streptokinase-Behandlung, *Thrombos. Diathes. Haemorrh. (Stuttg.),* 22, 121, 1969.
8. **Martin, M.,** Indirect measurement of streptokinase concentration in the plasma of patients undergoing fibrinolytic treatment, *Thrombos. Diathes. Haemorrh. (Stuttg.),* 32, 633, 1974.
9. **Martin, M.,** On the reliability of plasminogen measurement employing the proactivator-activator converting method, *Thrombos. Diathes. Haemorrh. (Stuttg.),* 36, 551, 1976.
10. **Lassen, M.,** Heat denaturization of plasminogen in the fibrin plate method, *Acta Phys. Scand.,* 27, 371, 1952.
11. **Martin, M.,** Quantitative streptokinase determination in plasma of patients undergoing thrombolytic therapy, *Semin. Thrombos. Hemost.,* 2, 33, 1975.
12. **Gram, H. C.,** A new method for determination of the fibrin percentage in blood and plasma, *J. Biol. Chem.,* 49, 279, 1921.
13. **Schulz, F. H.,** Eine einfache volumetrische Fibrin bestimmung, *Ärztl. Lab.,* 1, 107, 1955.
14. **Clauss, A.,** Gerinnungsphysiologische Schnellmethode zur Bestimmung des Fibrinogens, *Acta Haematol.,* 17, 237, 1957.
15. **Proctor, R. R. and Rapaport, S. J.,** The partial thromboplastin time with kaolin. A simple screening test for first stage plasma clotting factor deficiencies, *Am. J. Clin. Pathol.,* 36, 212, 1961.
16. **Jim, R. T. S.,** A study of the plasma thrombin time, *J. Lab. Clin. Med.,* 50, 45, 1957.
17. **Soria, J., Soria, C., Yver, J., and Samama, M.,** Temps de reptilase. Etude de la polymerisation de la fibrine en présence de reptilase, *Coagulation,* 2, 173, 1969.

Appendix

APPENDIX
(ANGIOGRAMS)

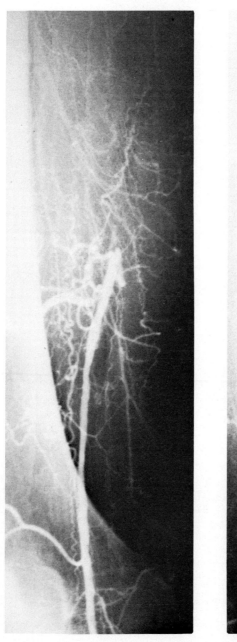 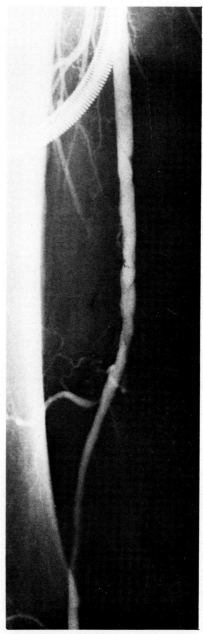

A   B

FIGURE A-1. Dissolution of a right femoral occlusion by streptokinase therapy. Occlusion age approximately 10 months. (A) Pretreatment angiogram. (B) Posttreatment angiogram. Vessel found still open at last recheck investigation 4 years 2 months later. Ref. No. 4.

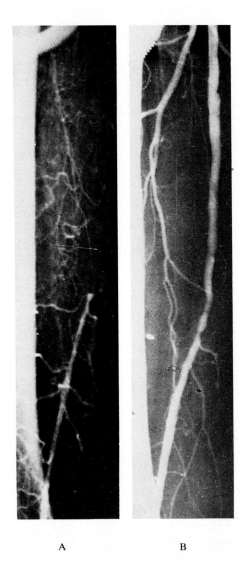

A   B

FIGURE A-2.   Dissolution of a right femoral occlusion by streptokinase therapy. Occlusion age approximately 4 weeks. (A) Pretreatment angiogram.
(B) Posttreatment angiogram. Note the persisting
anular stenosis in the distal portion of the cleared
segment. Vessel found still open at last recheck investigation 6 years 5 months later. Ref. No. 165.

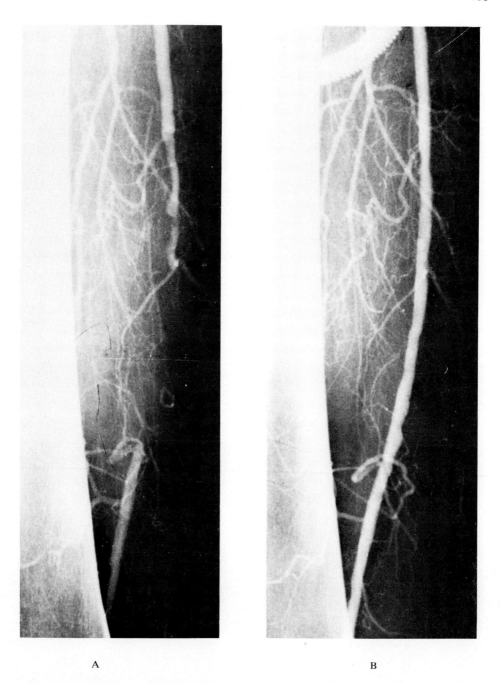

A B

FIGURE A-3. Dissolution of a right femoral occlusion by streptokinase therapy. Occlusion age approximately 2 weeks. (A) Pretreatment angiogram. (B) Posttreatment angiogram. Vessel still open at last recheck investigation 3 months later. Ref. No. 176.

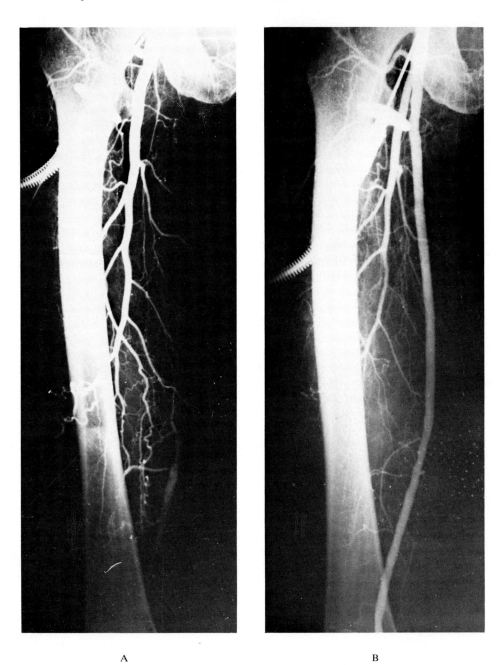

A   B

FIGURE A-4.   Dissolution of a right femoral occlusion by streptokinase therapy. Occlusion age approximately 4 weeks. (A) Pretreatment angiogram. (B) Posttreatment angiogram. Ref. No. B 1.

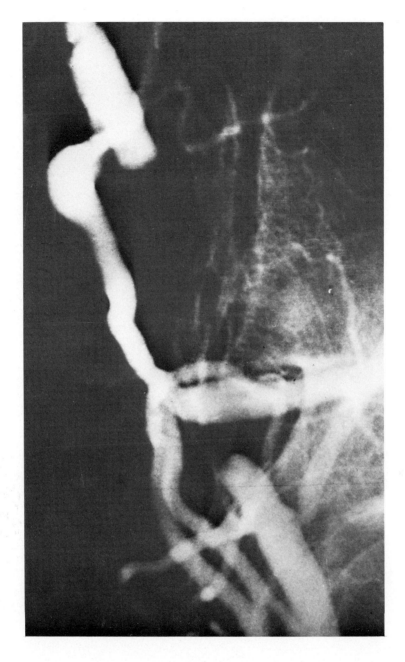

A

FIGURE A-5.   Dissolution of a left external iliac artery occlusion by streptokinase treatment. Occlusion age approximately 8 months. (A) Pretreatment angiogram. (B) Posttreatment angiogram. Ref. No. 143.

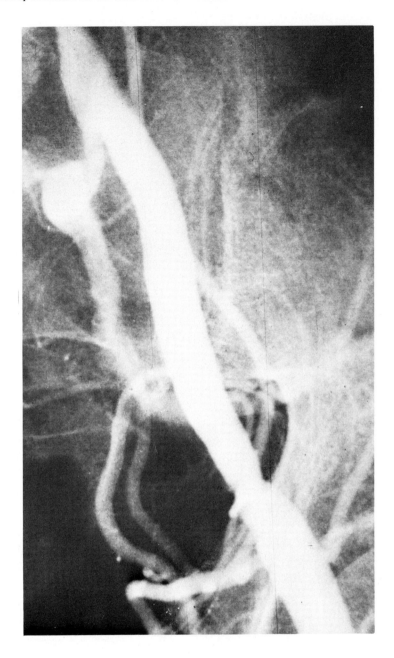

FIGURE A-5B.

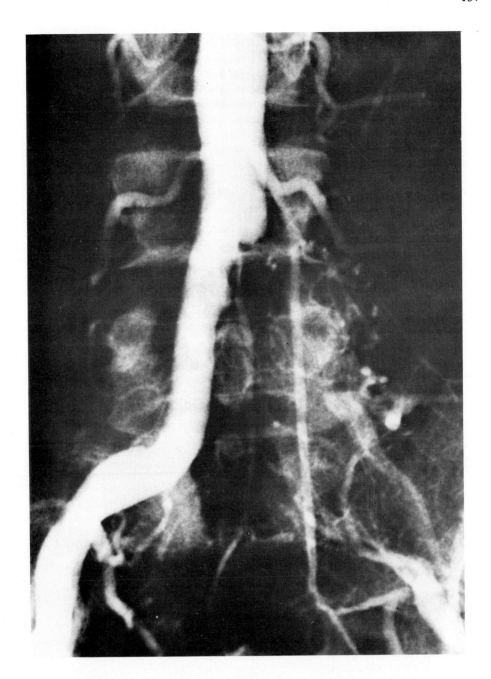

A

FIGURE A-6.   Dissolution of a left common iliac occlusion by streptokinase treatment. Occlusion age unknown. (A) Pretreatment angiogram. (B) Posttreatment angiogram shows clearance of the vessel with a persistent stenosis at the lower third part of the common iliac artery. (C) Recheck angiogram 14 months later demonstrates that the vessel is still open. (From Martin, M., *Progr. Cardiovasc. Dis.*, 21, 5, 1979. With permission.)

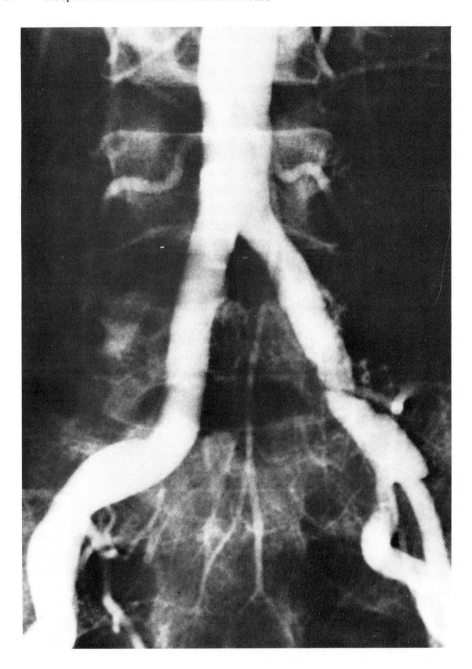

FIGURE A-6B.

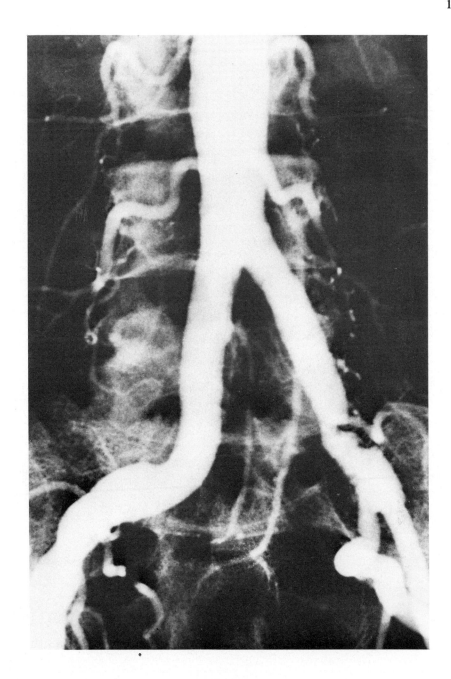

FIGURE A-6C.

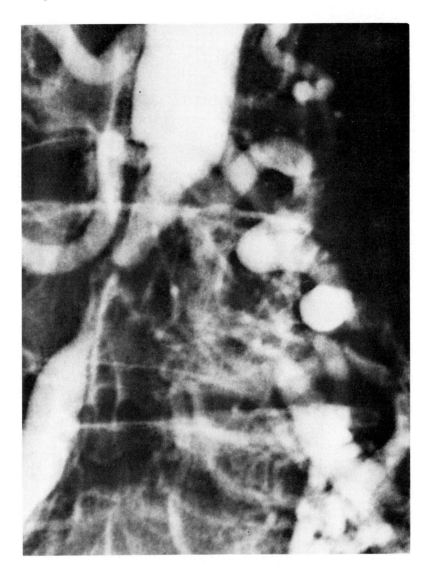

A

FIGURE A-7.   Dissolution of a left common iliac occlusion by streptokinase treatment.
Occlusion age unknown. (A) Pretreatment angiogram. (B) Posttreatment angiogram. The
formerly occluded segment is cleared but displays distinct narrowings. Seventeen days after
conducting the follow-up angiogram, reocclusion of the artery occurred. Ref. No. 83.

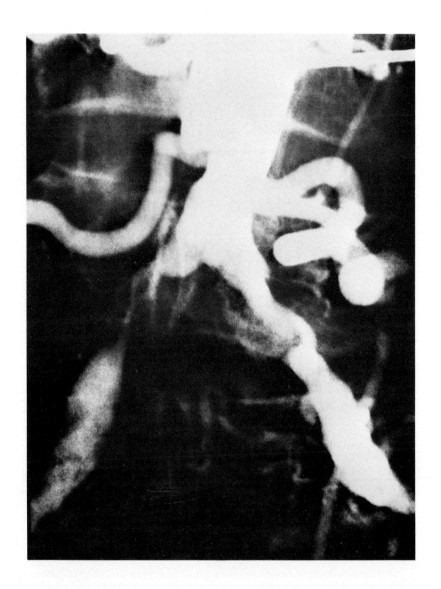

B.

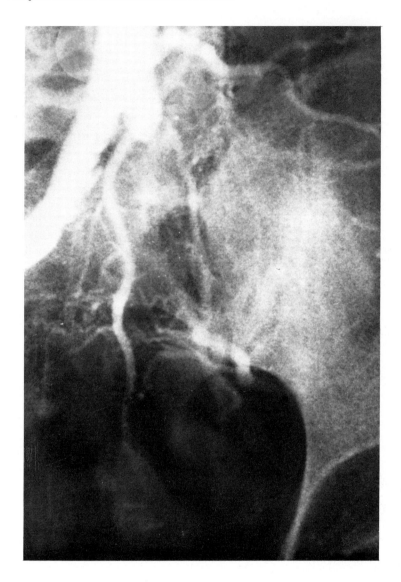

A

FIGURE A-8.   Dissolution of a left common iliac artery occlusion by streptokinase therapy. Occlusion age approximately 6 months. (A) Pretreatment angiogram. (B) Posttreatment angiogram. Vessel found still open at last recheck investigation 3 years 11 months later. Ref. No. 344.

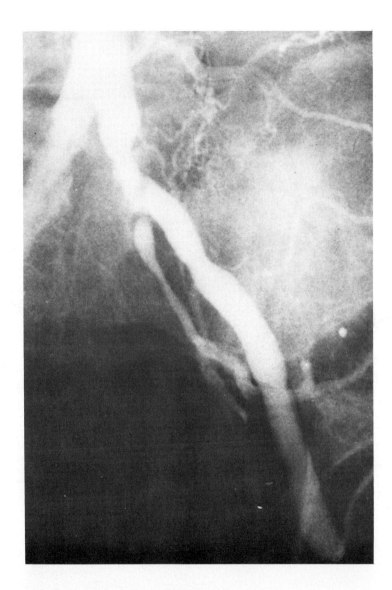

B

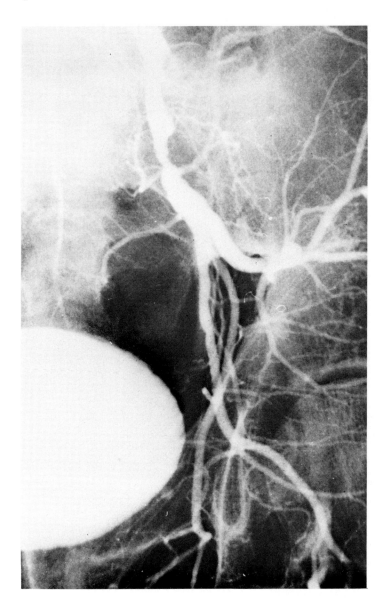

A

FIGURE A-9.   Dissolution of a left external iliac occlusion by streptokinase therapy. Occlusion age approximately 5 months. (A) Pretreatment angiogram. (B) Posttreatment. The formerly occluded segment is patent but narrowed extensively over a length of 2 cm. After a period of 2 months the vessel was still open. Subsequently, the residual stenosis was dilated by transluminal catheter technique. Ref. No. 401.

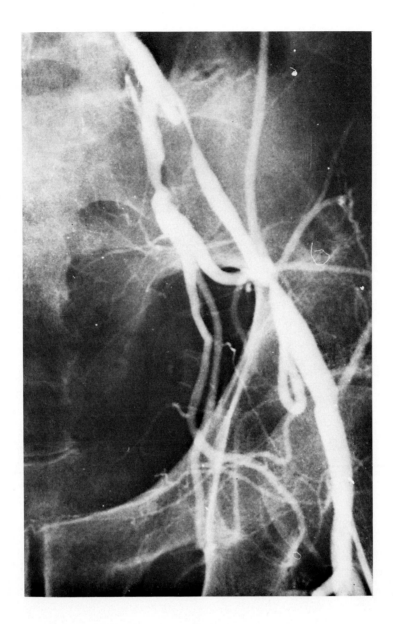

B

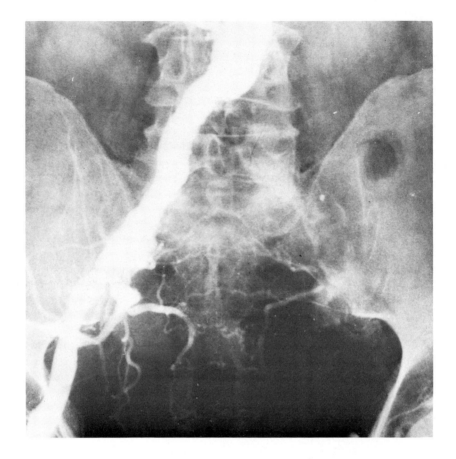

A

FIGURE A-10.   Dissolution of a left common iliac occlusion by streptokinase treatment. Occlusion age approximately 1 year. (A) Pretreatment angiogram. (B) Posttreatment angiogram. Vessel found still open at last recheck examination 1 year 10 months later. (From Martin, M., *Progr. Cardiovasc. Dis.,* 21, 5, 1979. With permission.)

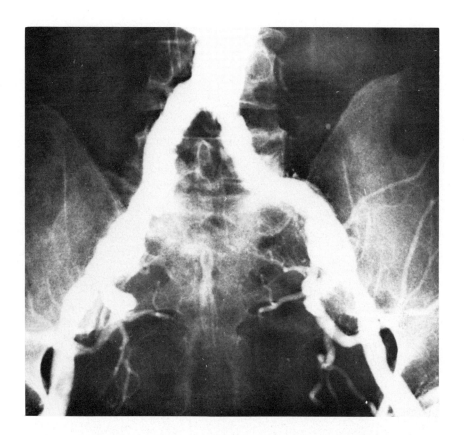

B

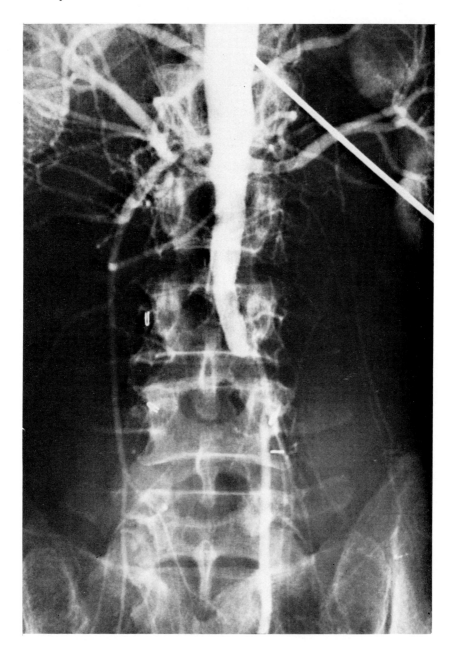

A

FIGURE A-11.   Dissolution of an aortic and right common iliac occlusion by streptokinase treatment. Occlusion age approximately 7 years. (A) Pretreatment angiogram. (B) Posttreatment angiogram. The formerly occluded left common iliac artery did not respond to treatment. The distal aorta and right common iliac artery was cleared. Despite a residual high grade anular stenosis on the distal part of the right common iliac artery (arrow), the vessels were found patent 11 months later. The patient died 1 year thereafter from acute heart failure. (From Martin, M., *Progr. Cardiovasc. Dis.*, 21, 5, 1979. With permission.)

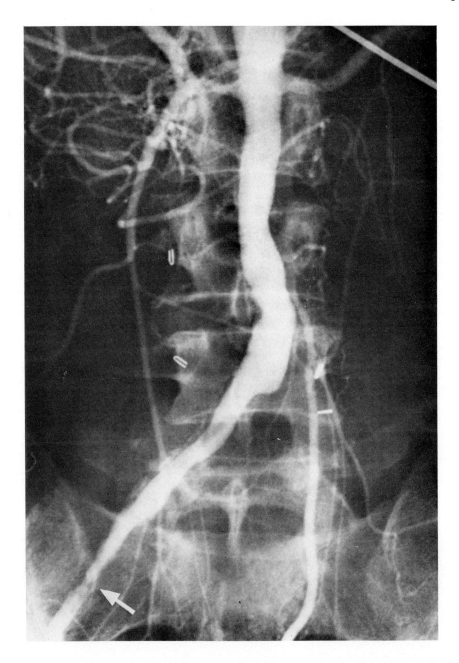

B

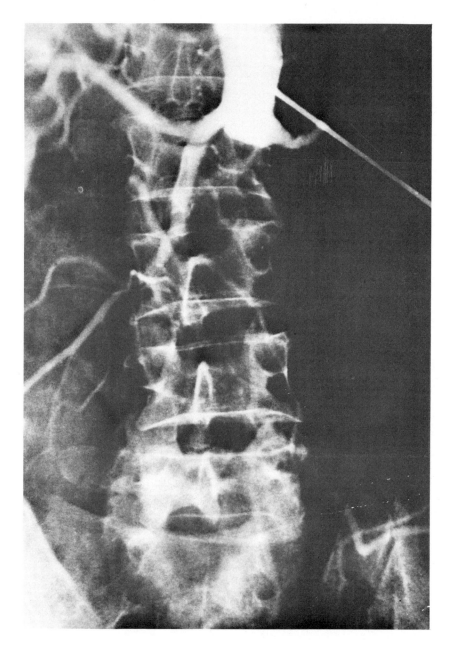

A

FIGURE A-12.   Dissolution of an aortic and bilateral common iliac occlusion by streptokinase treatment. Occlusion age approximately 7 years. (A) Pretreatment angiogram 1 year before lysis. (B) Pretreatment angiogram 2 weeks before lysis. (C) Posttreatment angiogram 2 weeks after concluding streptokinase therapy. With the exception of several band-like narrowings, aorta and iliac arteries were cleared. Reocclusion of the aorta occurred 3 years later. (From Martin, M., Schoop, W., and Zeitler, E., *JAMA,* 211, 1973. With permission.)

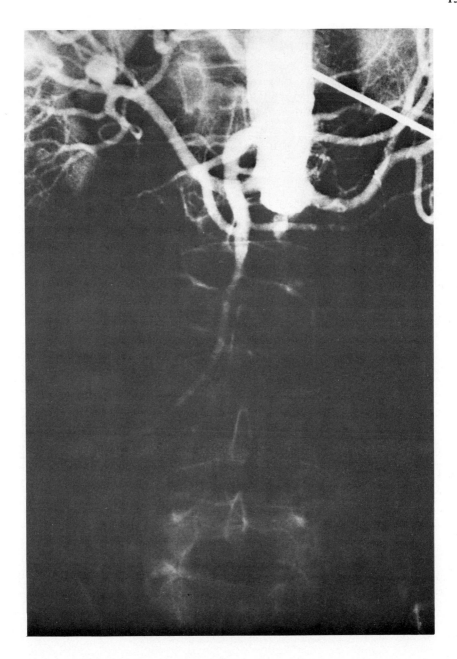

B

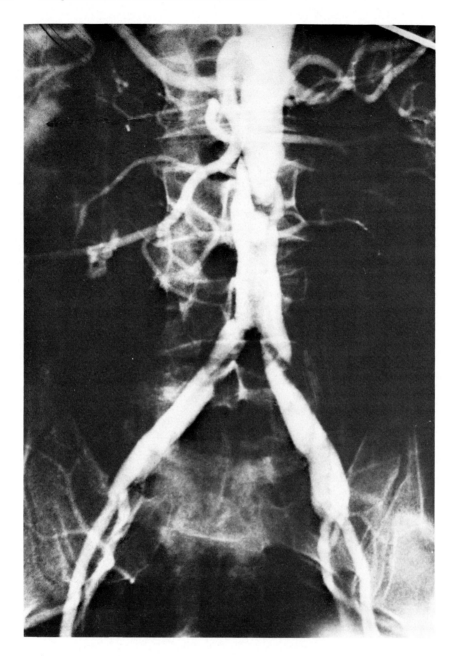

FIGURE A-12C.

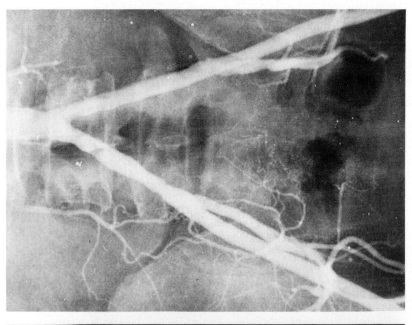

B

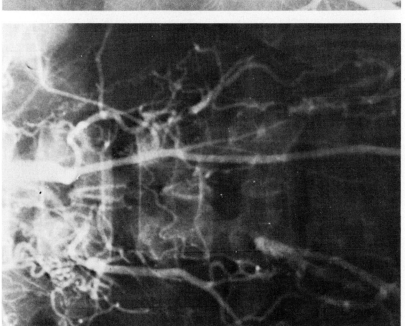

A

FIGURE A-13. Dissolution of an aortic and bilateral common iliac occlusion by streptokinase treatment. Occlusion age about 3 months. (A) Pretreatment angiogram. (B) Posttreatment angiogram. (C) Recheck angiogram showing the still patent vessel 3 years later. (From Martin, M., *Progr. Cardiovasc. Dis.*, 21, 5, 1979. With permission.)

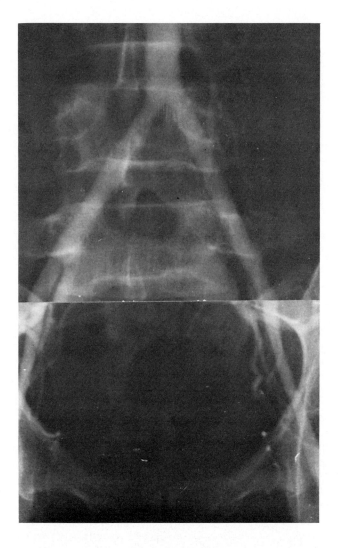

FIGURE A-13C

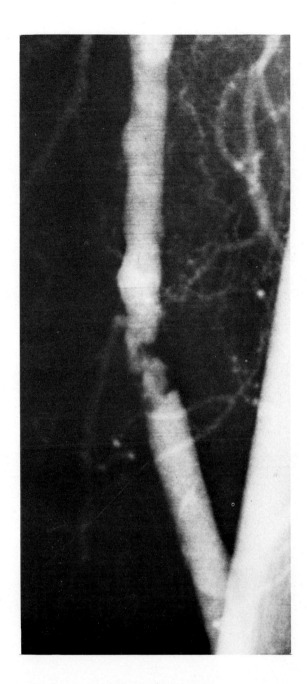

A

FIGURE A-14.   Widening of a left sided femoral stenosis. (A) Pretreatment angiogram showing a stenosis of Type A (see Chapter 10, Figure 1). (B) Posttreatment angiogram. Ref. No. 170.

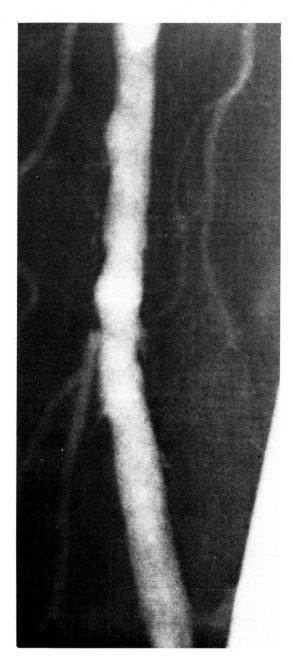

FIGURE A-14B

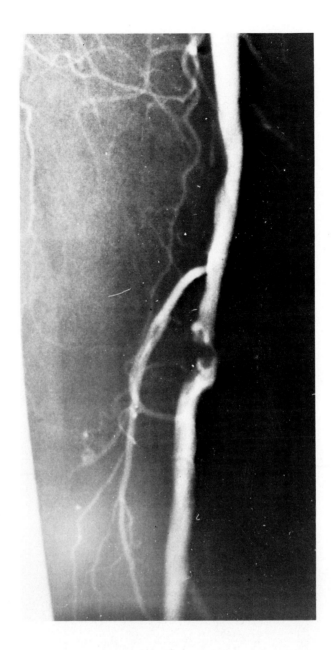

A

FIGURE A-15. Widening of a right sided femoral stenosis. (A) Pretreatment angiogram showing a narrowing of Type F (see Chapter 10, Figure 1). (B) Posttreatment angiogram. Ref. No. 303.

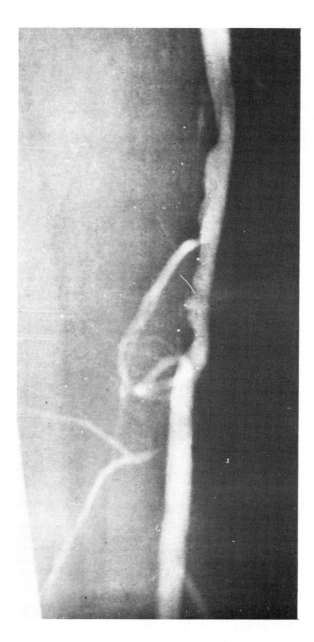

FIGURE A-15B.

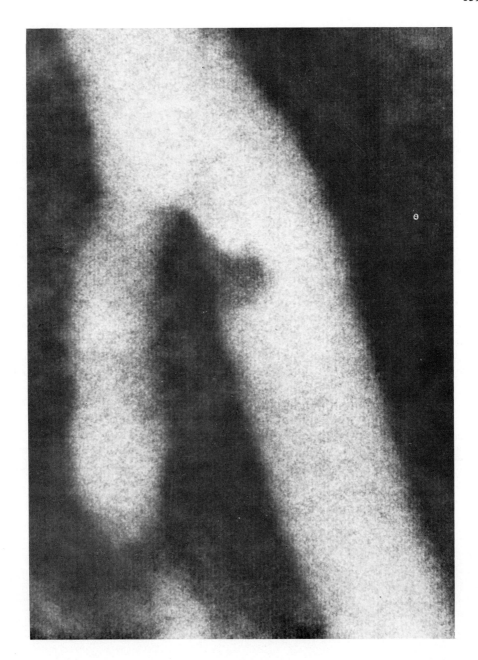

A

FIGURE A-16.   Dissolution of a thrombotic apposition adherent to the inner surface of the left external iliac artery. (A) Pretreatment angiogram showing the narrowing coded as Type R (see Chapter 10, Figure 1). (B) Posttreatment angiogram. Ref. No. 36.

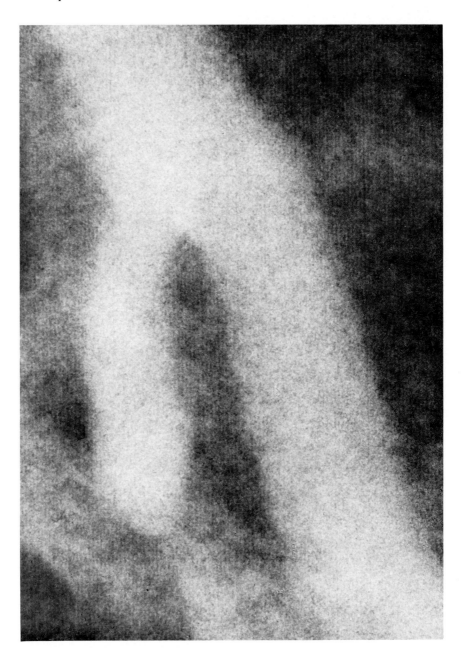

FIGURE A-16B.

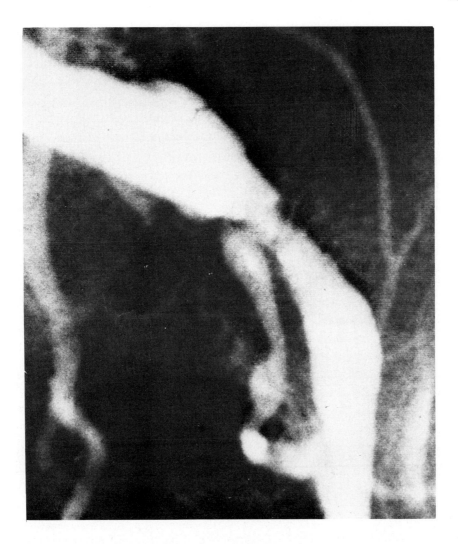

A

FIGURE A-17. Widening of a stenosis constricting the proximal portion of the left external iliac artery immediately behind the branching of the internal iliac artery. (A) Pretreatment angiogram showing the narrowing coded as Type D (see Chaper 10, Figure 1). (B) Posttreatment angiogram. Ref. No. 47.

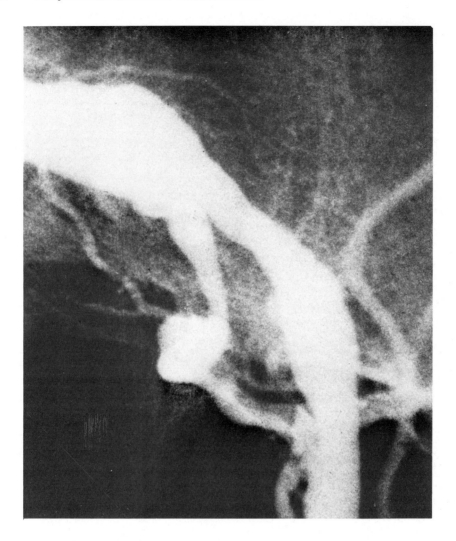

FIGURE A-17B.

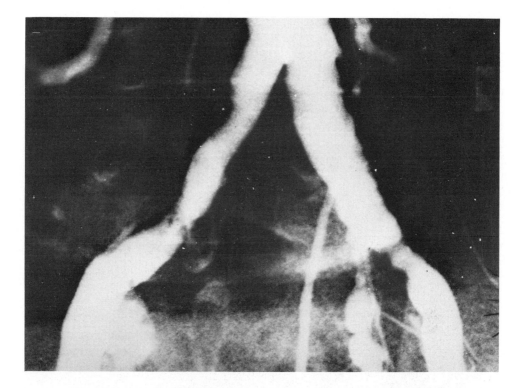

A

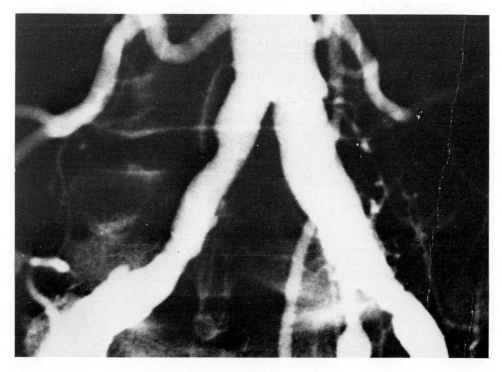

B

FIGURE A-18.   Widening of a stenosis located in the distal part of the right external iliac artery. (A) Pretreatment angiogram showing the narrowing coded as Type A (see Chapter 10, Figure 1). (B) Posttreatment angiogram. Ref. No. 57.

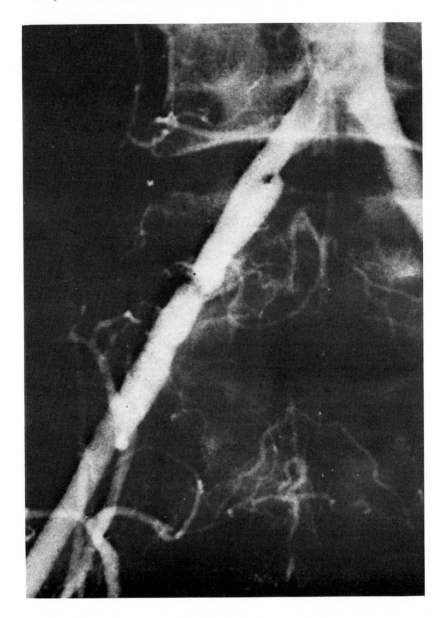

A

FIGURE A-19.   Widening of a stenosis located in the middle part of the right common iliac artery. (A) Pretreatment angiogram showing the narrowing coded as Type A (see Chapter 10, Figure 1). (B) Posttreatment angiogram. Ref. No. 70.

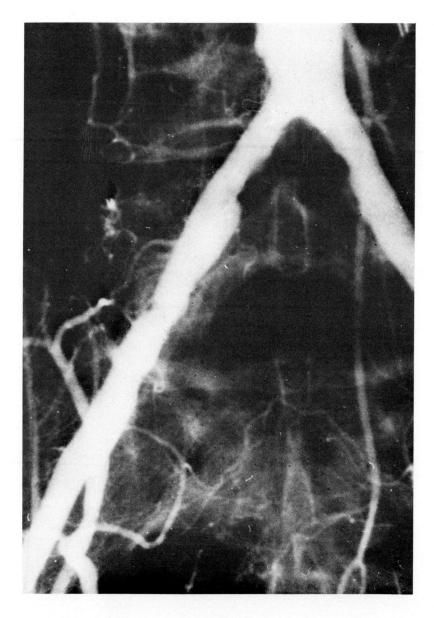

B

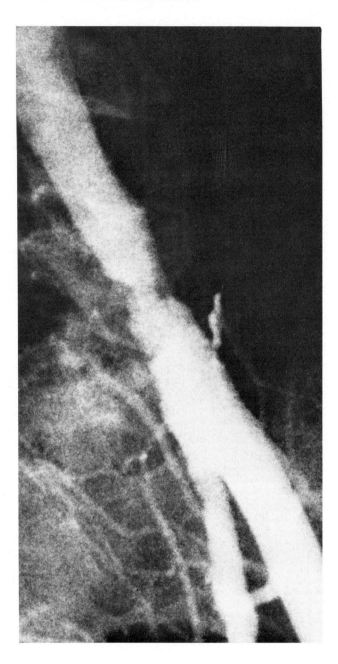

A

FIGURE A-20.   Widening of a stenosis located in the middle section
of the left common iliac artery. (A) Pretreatment angiogram showing
a narrowing coded as Type A (see Chapter 10, Figure 1). (B) Posttreatment angiogram. Ref. No. 64.

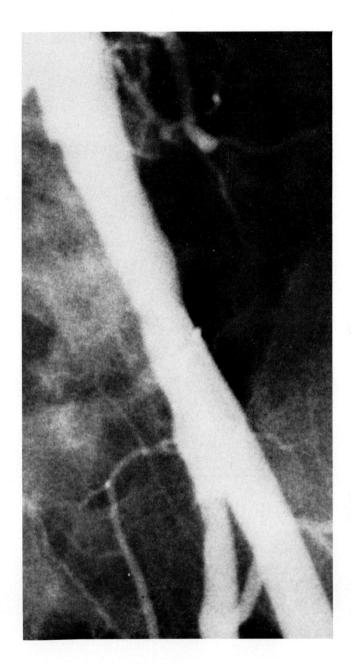

B

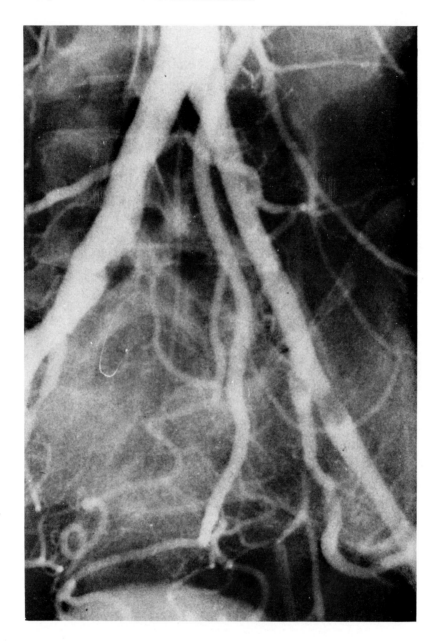

A

FIGURE A-21.   Widening of a stenosis located in the proximal part of the left external iliac artery. (A) Pretreatment angiogram showing the narrowing coded as Type K (see Chapter 10, Figure 1). (B) Posttreatment angiogram. Ref. No. 303.

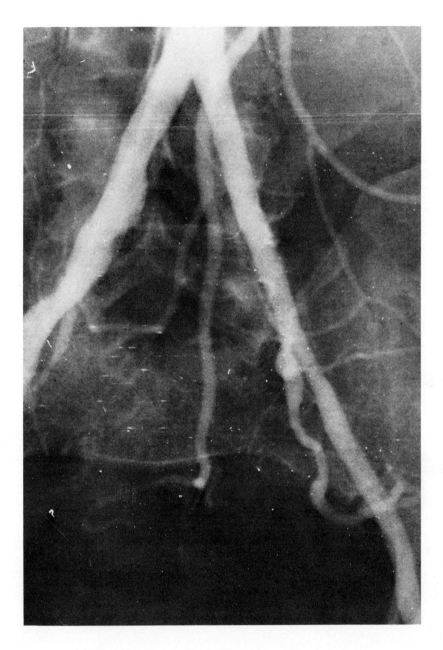

B

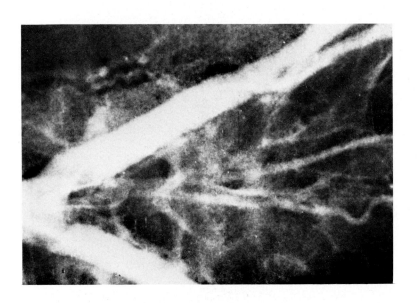

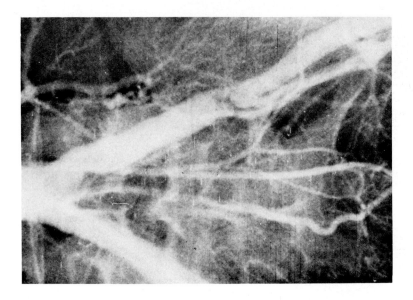

FIGURE A-22.   Widening of a stenosis located in the distal part of the left common iliac artery. (A) Pretreatment angiogram showing the narrowing coded as Type B (see Chapter 10, Figure 1). (B) Posttreatment angiogram. Ref. No. 319.

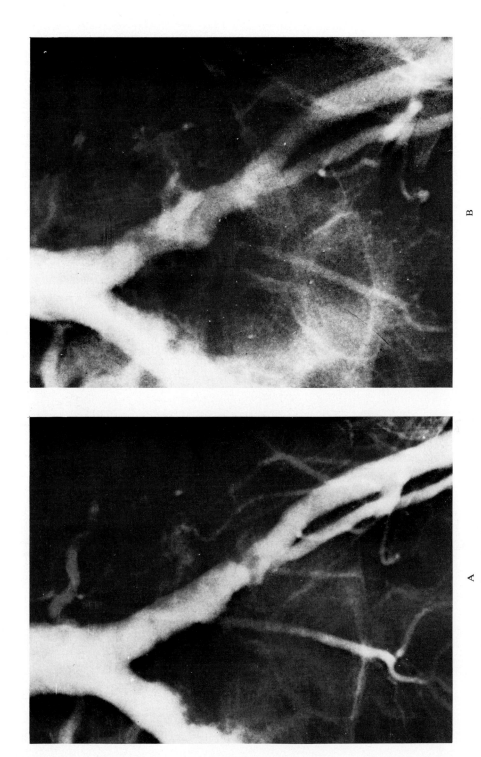

B

A

FIGURE A-23. Widening of a stenosis located in the distal third part of the left common iliac artery. (A) Pretreatment angiogram showing the narrowing coded as Type C (see Chapter 10, Figure 1). (B) Posttreatment angiogram. Ref. No. 444.

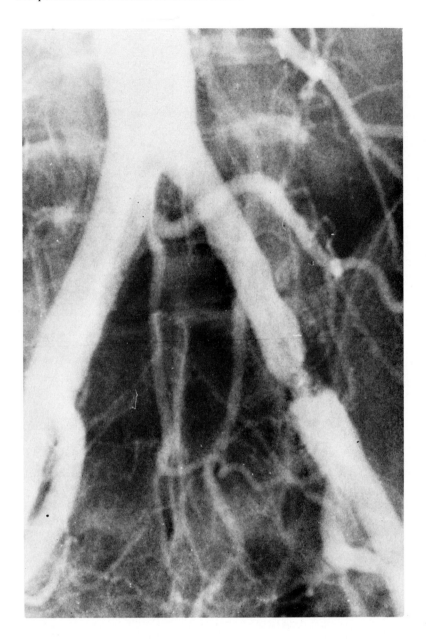

A

FIGURE A-24.   Widening of a stenosis located in the distal third part of the left common iliac artery. (A) Pretreatment angiogram showing the narrowing coded as Type A (see Chapter 10, Figure 1). (B) Posttreatment angiogram. Ref. No. 491.

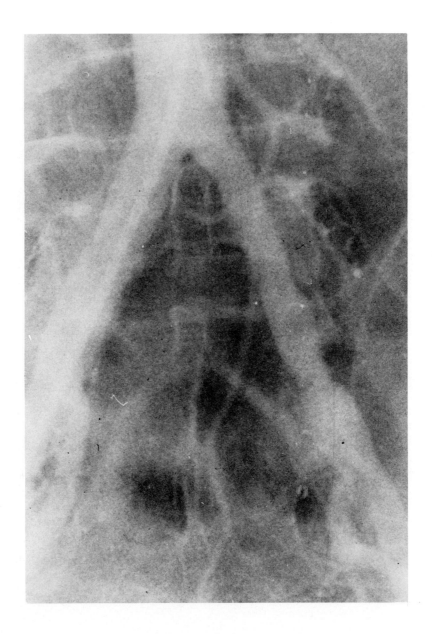

B

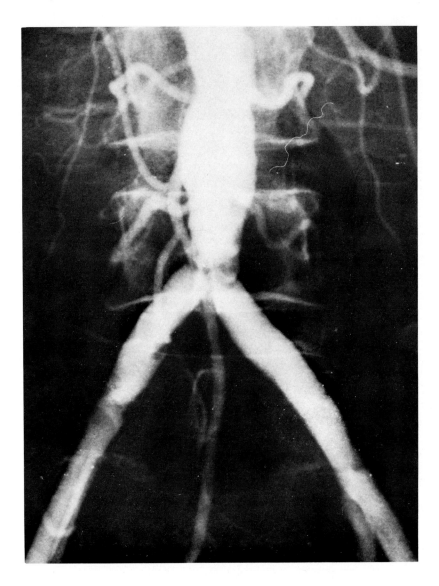

A

FIGURE A-25.   Widening of a stenosis located around the aortic bifurcation. (A) Pretreatment angiogram showing the narrowing coded as Type A (see Chapter 10, Figure 1).
(B) Posttreatment angiogram. Ref. No. 86.

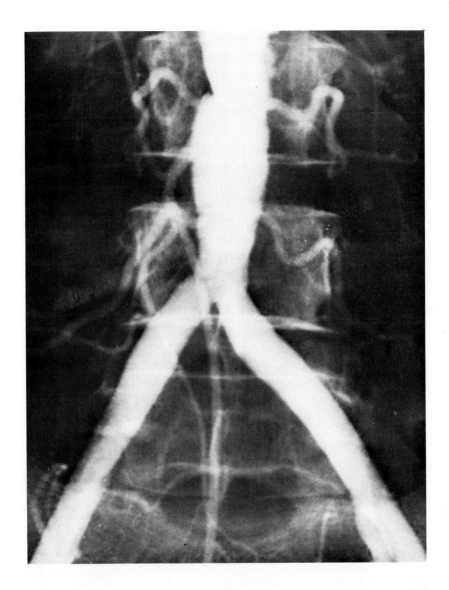

B

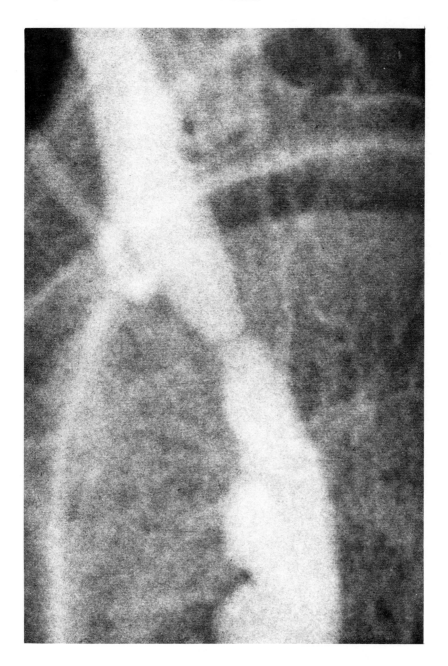

FIGURE A-26.   Angiographic representation of an arterial stenosis (located in the left external iliac artery) coded as Type M2 (Ref. No. 115). According to current experience, no lytic widening is possible in this type of anular constriction. For more details, see Chapter 10.

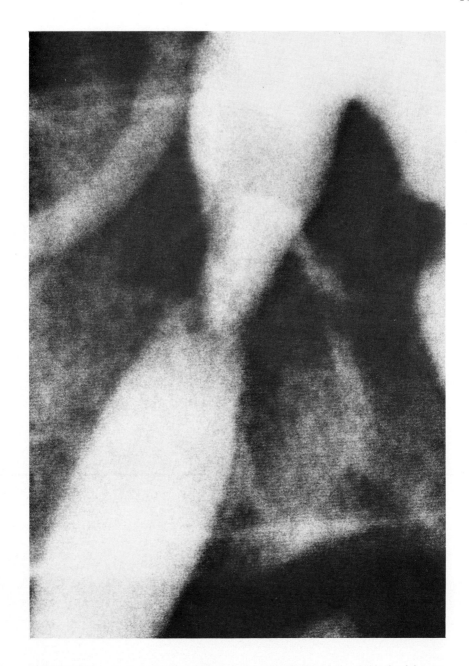

FIGURE A-27.   Angiographic representation of an arterial stenosis (located in the right common iliac artery) coded as Type M3 (Ref. No. 131). According to current experience, no lytic widening can be expected in this kind of smooth, hourglass formed narrowing. For more details, see Chapter 10.

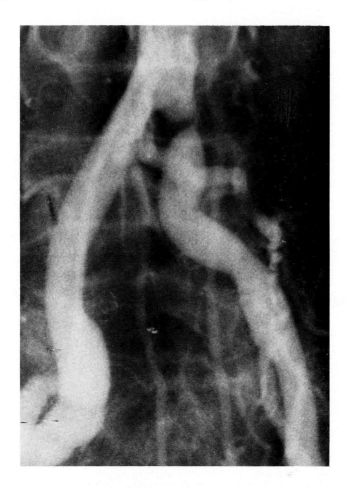

FIGURE A-28.   Angiographic representation of an arterial stenosis (located in the left common iliac artery) coded as Type M1 (Ref. No. 468). According to current experience, no lytic dilation is possible in this hourglass formed constriction. For more details, see Chapter 10. (From Martin, M., *Progr. Cardiovasc. Dis.*, 21, 5, 1979. With permission.)

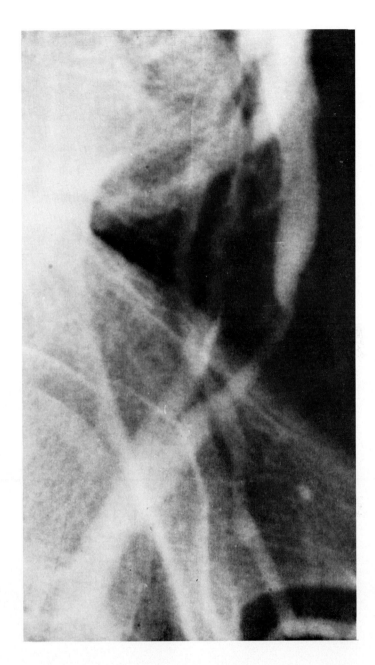

FIGURE A-29.   Angiographic representation of an arterial stenosis (located in the right external iliac artery) coded as Type P (Ref. No. 95). According to current experience, no lytic dilation is possible in this type of thread-like constriction. For more details see Chapter 10. (From Martin, M., *Progr. Cardiovasc. Dis.*, 21, 5, 1979. With permission.)

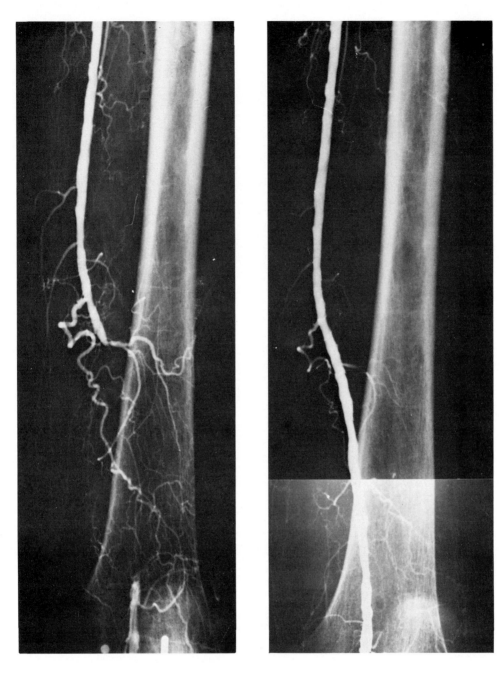

A   B

FIGURE A-30.   Removal of a left femoral arterial occlusion located in the lower third segment by catheter lysis procedure. Occlusion age approximately 2 months. (A) Pretreatment angiogram. (B) Posttreatment angiogram with vessel almost completely cleared. Ref. No. 495.

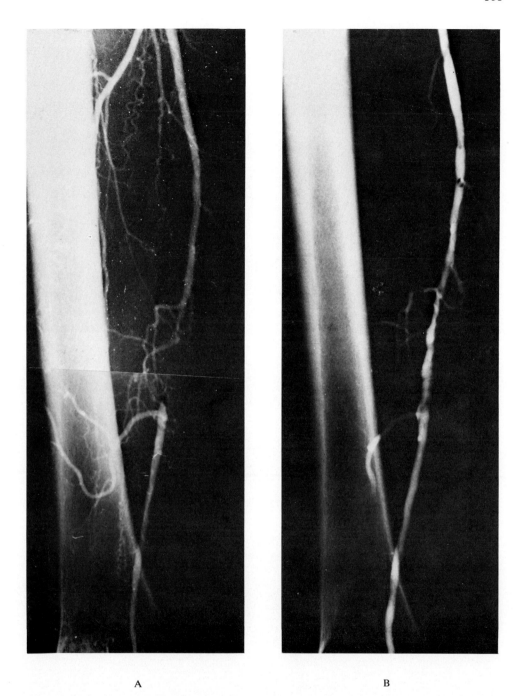

A　　　　　　　　　　　　B

FIGURE A-31.   Removal of a right femoral arterial occlusion located in the middle part of the vessel by catheter lysis procedure. Occlusion age approximately 6 months. (A) Pretreatment angiogram. (B) Post-trreatment angiogram. The vessel is cleared, but with multiple stenoses remaining. Ref. no. 488.

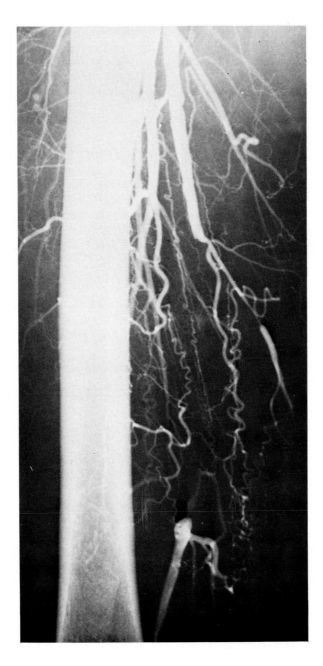

A

FIGURE A-32.   Removal of a right femoral occlusion by the catheter lysis procedure. Occlusion age approximately 6 months. (A) Pretreatment angiogram. (B) Postlysis angiogram with a residual stenosis at the distal end of the formerly occluded segment. (C) State after dilating the residual stenosis by Dotter's transluminal catheter technique. Ref. No. 485.

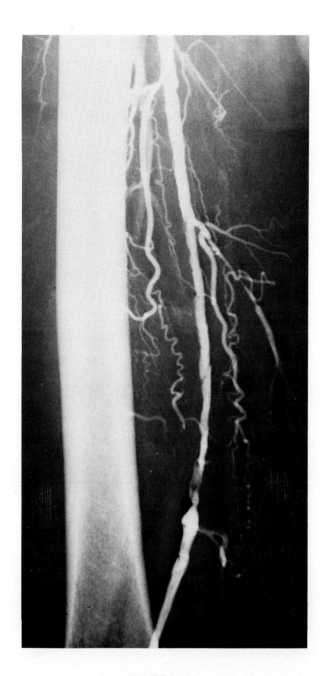

FIGURE A-32B.

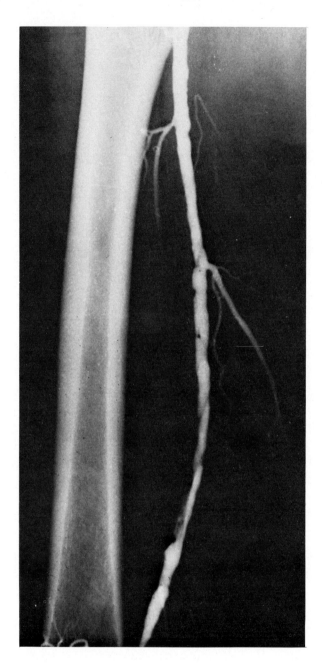

FIGURE A-32C.

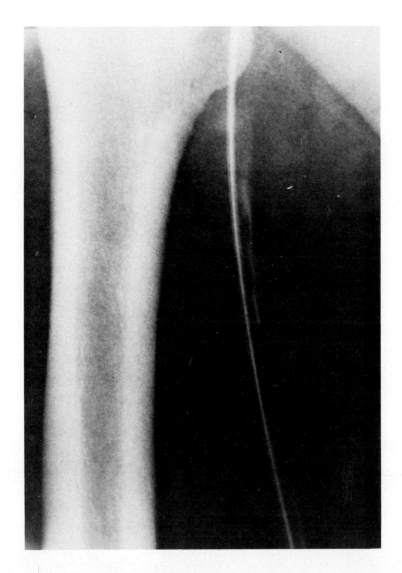

FIGURE A-33.   Thrombic material adherent to the surface of a catheter after 24 hr of catheter lysis procedure. The catheter tip (not shown on this angiogram) was placed in the midst of the thrombus material, building up a femoral occlusion. By removing the catheter, the adhering material was wiped off and remained in the vessel.

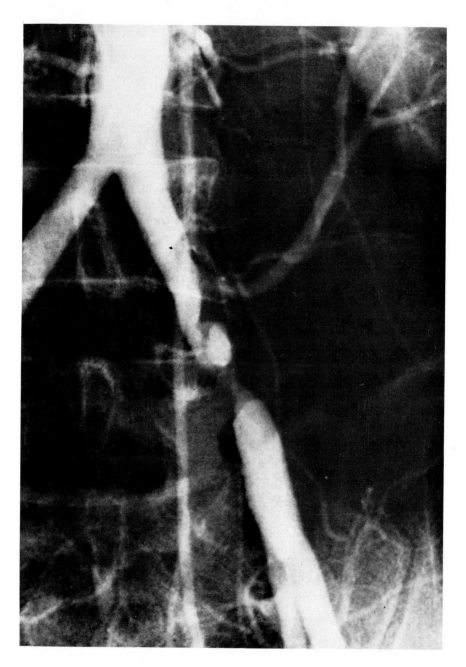

A

FIGURE A-34.   Angiographic demonstration of both a fibrinolytic success and a newly formed thrombotic apposition. (A) The angiogram shows two subsequent narrowings in the middle part of the left common iliac artery just beneath the branching of an aberrant left renal artery. (B) Angiogram after streptokinase treatment. The proximal stenosis has vanished but the distal one shows a significant deterioration (extension into the distal direction, higher grade of constriction). Ref. No. 103.

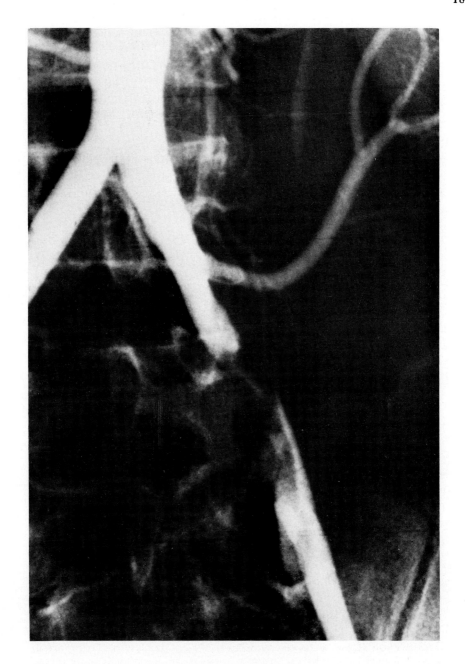

FIGURE A-34B.

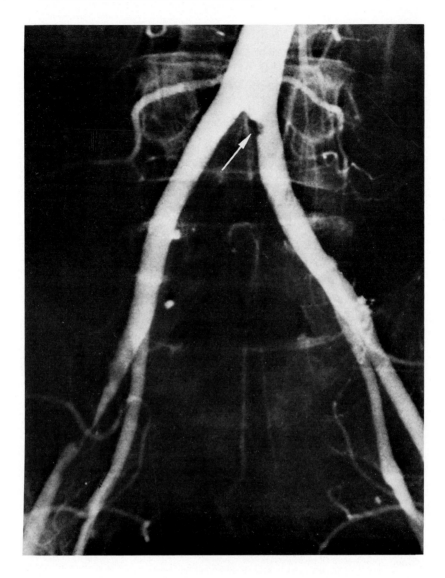

A

FIGURE A-35.   Angiographic demonstration of both a fibrinolytic success and a newly formed thrombotic occlusion. (A) The angiogram shows a thrombotic apposition on the proximal part of the left common iliac artery, plus a high grade, thread-like stenosis of the right external iliac artery. (B) After streptokinase therapy, the left sided apposition has vanished, whereas the right stenosis has been transformed into a complete occlusion. Ref. No. 87.

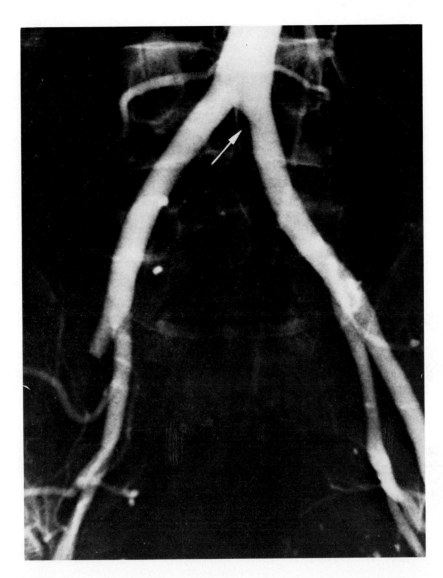

FIGURE A-35B.

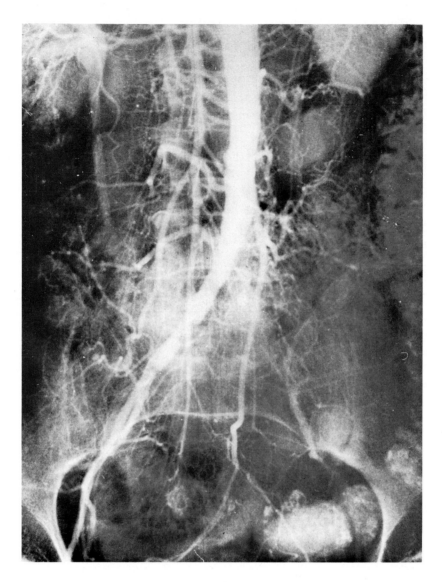

A

FIGURE A-36. Demonstration of a thrombotic aortic occlusion following streptokinase treatment. (A) Pretreatment angiogram shows a common iliac stenosis on the right side and a common, as well as an external iliac occlusion, on the left side. (B) Posttreatment angiogram. Thrombotic masses have developed in the lumen of the abdominal aorta, nearly occluding the vessel. This was confirmed by vascular surgery. The occlusion settled during the week following streptokinase treatment. No anticoagulants were given over that period of time. Ref. No. 100.

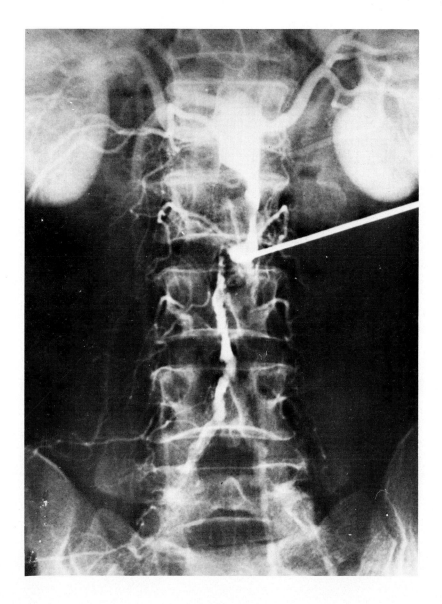

FIGURE A-36B.

INDEX